The Complete Guide to Walking
for Health, Weight Loss, and Fitness
New and Revised

Mark Fenton

The Lyons Press
Guilford, Connecticut
An imprint of The Globe Pequot Press

The health information expressed in this book is based solely on the personal experience of the author and is not intended as a medical manual. The information should not be used for diagnosis or treatment, or as a substitute for professional medical care. The author and publisher urge you to consult with your health care provider prior to beginning any exercise program.

Copyright © 2001, 2008 by R. D. Walking, Inc.

ALL RIGHTS RESERVED. No part of this book may be reproduced or transmitted in any form by any means, electronic or mechanical, including photocopying and recording, or by any information storage and retrieval system, except as may be expressly permitted in writing from the publisher. Requests for permission should be addressed to The Globe Pequot Press, Attn: Rights and Permissions Department, P.O. Box 480, Guilford, CT 06437.

The Lyons Press is an imprint of The Globe Pequot Press.

PHOTO CREDITS

David Roth: 4, 10, 19, 29, 33, 39, 41, 42, 43, 62, 66, 91, 95, 103, 123, 128, 139, 163, 170, 204, 225, 227, 228; Keller & Keller: 6, 7, 115, 116, 117, 118, 125 (bottom), 164, 165, 166, 167, 168; David Tsay: 14, 54, 75, 97, 130, 158, 175; Judith Broggi: 44, 45, 100, 101; Jim Janos: 196, 197; Carolyn Ros: 208, 209, 210; Furnald / Gray: 34, 159; Mark Fenton: x, xii, 189; Vito Aluia: 125 (top 4); Michael Lanza: 173; The Baby Jogger Company: 57; www.photos.com: 35, 102, 203; Leki Walking Poles: 120; Gary Higgins: 127, 223.

10 9 8 7 6 5 4 3 2 1

Printed in China

Designed by A Good Thing, Inc.

ISBN: 978-1-59228-989-9

The Library of Congress has previously cataloged an earlier edition as follows:

Fenton, Mark.
    Walking magazine's the complete guide to walking for health, weight loss, and fitness / Mark Fenton
        p. cm.
    Includes index.
    ISBN: 1-58574-190-6
    1. Fitness walking. 2. Weight loss. 3. Physical fitness. I. Title: The complete guide to walking for health, weight loss, and fitness. II. Walking magazine. III. Title.
RA 781.65.F646 2001
613.7'176—dc21   00-63104

Contents

Introduction

Two words: more walking

Since I first wrote this book I've had the good fortune to travel across North America as a "walking expert." I guess that's what happens when you write a "complete guide" to anything—you become an expert. My travels have taken me from launching fitness walking programs at work sites in Palo Alto, California, to working with planners designing a better pedestrian and bicycle network in Charlotte, North Carolina. I've spoken to trail advocates in Portland, Oregon, and the health insurance industry in Portland, Maine. I've done health promotion and walkable community workshops across the plains of Saskatchewan, Canada, and worked with high school students to encourage healthy lifestyles in Nogales, Arizona, on the Mexican border. And the one theme—the one constant in all of my work—revolves around the two words that are the centerpiece of my recommendations for every community I visit. Those two words: More walking. Whether helping overweight people in a beginning fitness program or helping an employer lower his health care costs, the thread is to get folks to do more walking. Want to feel increased energy and less stress? Walk more. Looking to get folks shopping downtown? Make it appealing for walking. Need to lower those cholesterol and blood pressure numbers? Try a daily walk. Struggling to reduce traffic congestion and dump less carbon dioxide into the atmosphere? Get everyone to walk once a week instead of driving to work. I've had two personal experiences since writing the book that have reassured me how much everyone needs the simple prescription contained within these pages. They reconfirmed for me that more walking really is the answer for individuals, families, and even entire communities.

Confirmation number one

Just over a year ago a crazy friend of mine started hounding me about an idea he had to hike the famed John Muir Trail (JMT) in the Sierra Nevada Mountains of California. This trail is an icon of magnificence to backpackers nationwide, and each year many traverse its 220 miles stretching from Yosemite National Park in the north to Mt. Whitney in the south. Simply put, this is the country that inspired Muir to embark on his successful advocacy for a National Park system.

So, if it's such a beautiful, classic hike, why was it such a crazy idea to tackle it? Because most people plan two to three weeks averaging 10 to 15 miles a day. They also carry 50 to 60 pound packs, especially near the beginning of the hike when laden with the most food. But my friend Mike Lanza, an editor at *Backpacker* magazine who has clearly suffered too much oxygen deprivation at high altitudes, had another idea entirely. He wanted to try out the latest gear—ultralight packs, sleeping bags, tarps, and clothes all designed for minimalist, high-speed hiking. His clever notion was that with super light packs maxing out at 25 pounds, we'd be able to hike so fast we wouldn't need three weeks worth of food (making the packs even lighter) and thus we'd be able to cover the full trek in *seven* days. That's 31 miles a day! I should have done the math and told Mike to stick some trail mix in his ear and leave me alone, but he eventually convinced me, and a late August date was set.

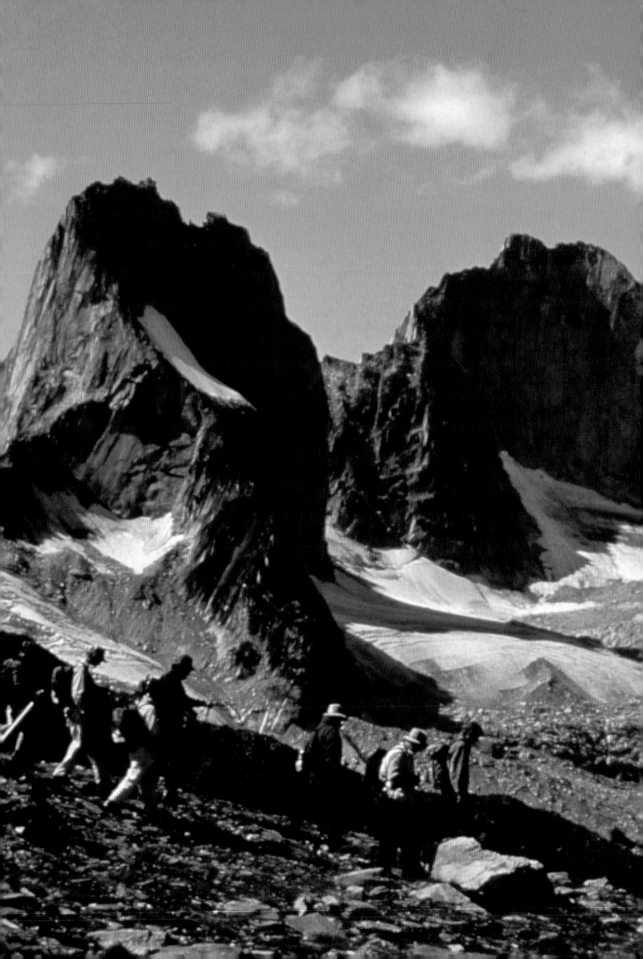

Here's the interesting thing—by the middle of the summer, I realized that the challenge might not be the hike itself, but getting in good enough shape while living a real life with a real family and work. But with Mike's cajoling I managed a series of great 4:00 a.m., 15 to 20 mile trail hikes on Saturdays (the early start assured I'd be home in time for soccer with the kids and dinner with my lovely bride) plus multiple shorter but speedy mid-week walks to build aerobic fitness. In other words, I found a way to build an intense walking training program into my busy weeks, and get into trail-ready shape by August.

The hike was one of the toughest things I've ever done, and I truly was ready to bail out on day five when one of our team had to hike out a side canyon due to toe-blisters the size of cocktail wieners. But thanks to great hiking partners I made it to the end of the trail in one, admittedly exhausted, piece. All it took on my part was *more walking*.

Confirmation number two

Several years ago I found myself at something of a mid-life crisis. I was leaving a job of many years at *WALKING* Magazine, beginning work on a new PBS television series (about walking), and writing another book (*Pedometer Walking*). Plus, we were sending our five-year-old son off to kindergarten and three-year-old daughter to preschool. Our babies were growing up, I was turning forty, and my career was decidedly, well, pedestrian.

My wife, Lisa, was getting nervous. She figured it was only a matter of time before I came home with a Gibson six string or Harley Davidson. So around my birthday in July, she took me out to our favorite local bistro for an "Of course we love the guy you've become" dinner. That talk-about-walking, eat-your-vegetables-and-be-healthy kind of guy. I was appreciative, but unconvinced I was really making a difference.

Returning to our neighborhood that evening we crossed a bridge that's a gentle arc over a tidal estuary. Sometimes the water's deep and swiftly flowing, sometimes a shallow trickle. As in many coastal towns (I've learned in my travels) it's a summer rite of passage for the local kids to jump off the bridge into the current. Of course, you've got to time the tide and depth right, or you can end up with feet sliced by razor-sharp barnacles. Or worse.

As it happened, two young girls in swimsuits were standing outside the rail of the bridge. They faced the water, but their arms were wrapped back over the railing in a serious grip; both looked nervous about jumping. I heard the voice of a teenage boy—not the apex of good human judgment—shouting up from the water below, "Go ahead, jump. It's deep enough, c'mon, let's go."

The girls responded, "Is it cold?"

"NO, just hurry up and jump."

"Why?"

Now, I didn't want to interrupt this intellectual dialogue, but what were Lisa and I supposed to do? Yell at them to get off the bridge? Or let kids be kids—just pass by and shake our heads?

So what do you think happened? Lisa looked at me and said, "Okay, give me your wallet, and take off that shirt. Go on, just be careful."

I handed her my wallet, pulled off my shirt and sandals, scrambled over the railing, and said, "Will you guys jump if I do?"

The girls were astonished. "Uh, yeah, I guess." And so jump we did—and safely swam to the other side.

Now, it was worth it just for the thrill of the jump, and for the looks on the kids' faces. ("The old fart's definitely going to die or explode or something when he hits the water.") But I've left the most important detail out of the story. How do you figure Lisa and I had traveled to dinner that evening? We'd walked, of course. We were passing those girls on foot, separated not by thousands of pounds of automotive steel and glass, but by just a short distance from the sidewalk to their precarious perch. And I could see in the girls' eyes that they were concerned—maybe it was their first jump, even. And in that moment, they were my kids. God forbid my wife and I woke the next morning and heard one had broken a leg. We had to stay and make sure they were safe, just as I hope someone else will do when my kids are old enough to be out on the bridge without me. We were there because of just two words: More walking.

As disconnected as they seem, these two stories illustrate the broad scope and vast positive impact of this most basic of human activities. On the surface, the first shows the vast health and fitness benefits of walking. With "mere" walking I was able to get in shape for a daunting 220-mile hike over rugged terrain, and at age forty be as fit as I've ever been in my life. That's saying something for a guy who tried out for two Olympic teams in the 50-kilometer racewalk in his twenties and thirties. It's proof that walking can get you to any fitness level you desire.

The second story, however, is just as important. Only because we were walking did Lisa and I interact with the bridge jumpers. Just as important, only because I walk all over my town did those kids recognize me and know me as a local, I hope allaying any concerns that I was some weirdo. It illustrates a greater truth—that more walking helps reconnect the social fabric of our communities. Those too young and too old to drive can still walk. Neighbors greet neighbors, streets feel safer, and local businesses thrive. There's less traffic, the air is cleaner, and we interact more when we do more walking.

How to use this book

This book is set up to help you learn, through experience, all of these lessons for yourself. My stories (and many others) confirm some of the basic lessons that you'll learn in this book about living an active lifestyle. I realized for myself once again that setting a goal and preparing for it is a powerful motivator. That having a plan (like the training program in here) vastly improves your likelihood of success, whether training for 220 miles of hiking or to lose 22 pounds.

During my training I experienced the protective power of proper, if brief and simple, daily warm-ups and cool-down stretches. Mike and I even took a few minutes for a handful of yoga stretches at the end of 15-hour hiking days. It certainly confirms the warm-ups and stretches in this book are worth your time.

I was reminded of the miraculous power of supportive friends and family, shown repeatedly in research to improve exercise adherence. On days five and seven of our hike, my colleagues were the difference between success and failure for me. This—called "social support" by researchers—and other proven motivational tips are presented throughout the book.

The value of the right gear was driven home—whether a two-pound sleeping bag rated for frigid mountain nights, or a decent pair of walking shoes for cruising around the neighborhood every morning.

Most important, I was reminded of the single greatest benefit of an active lifestyle: that it leaves the door open for adventures of every kind. Because in the end physical activity is its own reward. You don't have to do it to lose weight or reduce your risk for cardiovascular disease or Type II diabetes. It's not just so you fit in that specific outfit for your class reunion, or to keep your cholesterol number down. Do it because being active feels great, because it absolutely energizes you, because it gives you a feeling of accomplishment and being alive. Be a walker because you always feel better *after* a walk than you did before. (Yes, even a walk of 220 miles!) Be physically active because, to put it simply, it's fun!

To help you on your way to an active lifestyle, this book is disguised as an exercise guide. But it's really a user's manual for the human body. After all, read a few chapters of a book in 15 minutes, and burn about 15 calories; walk a mile in 15 minutes and you could burn over 100. So this is designed to have you reading and walking at the same time. After all, it's the walking, not the reading, that's gong to bring the results you're looking for. So read chapter one, then take the "Kick Off Your Walking" quiz, and jump right in to the accompanying one-year walking program.

As you progress through the one-year program certain questions about health, weight loss, technique, equipment, fitness and more will occur to you. The goal is that answers to all of these questions will always be right at your fingertips. Below are the six central lessons of this book. Once you've walked your way through these pages, you'll not only have learned these lessons, you'll have lived them.

You'll learn how to:
- Build a habit of daily walking and a lifestyle of greater physical activity.
- Target at least 30 minutes' worth of walking every day, weaving it into your daily routine whenever possible.
- Use every motivational trick you can to start, maintain, and return after a setback to your walking.
- Walk longer when you have the time.
- Walk faster (and use healthy technique) when you have less time or are looking for a more intense workout.
- Build elements of flexibility, strength, and coordination into your healthy lifestyle.

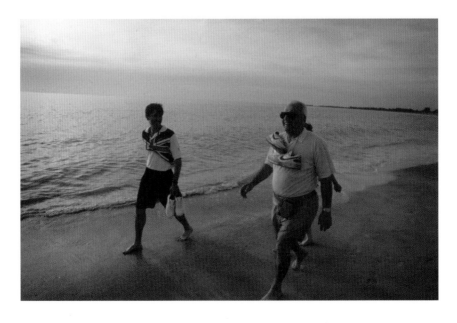

The program in this book is one year long for a reason. You started life as a kid being active—crawling, climbing, running around, chasing, and generally having to be told to sit still while you ate, got a haircut, or did some other unnaturally sedentary thing. Then over the next twenty years you learned how to be quiet and behave, listen in class and not squirm. Next thing you knew, you didn't have twenty minutes in your day for exercise.

My point is you didn't learn to be sedentary all at once and you won't become active again all at once either. The book is organized to get you moving in the same way you stopped—gradually, in bite-size pieces.

	What you get:	The Program:
Part I	Health and well-being. The basics of moving a little more every day.	16 weeks to averaging a 30-minute daily walk.
Part II	Weight loss or control. Longer walks for more calorie burning, and venturing off-road for more fun.	16 weeks to build the length of your walks, and prepare you for an all-day hike.
Part III	Total fitness and strength. Faster walks and a complete exercise program to build total fitness.	16 weeks of building intensity and preparing for a formal walking event.
Part IV	Lifelong Fitness. Making your personal plan for a lifetime of healthy activity.	4 weeks to act as your template, with lots of workout and motivational ideas.

Put it all together and you've got a one-year walking program. The program pages are numbered by week and bordered in color so they're easy to find. There's space for you to write what you've done each day, to act as your training log. If you don't want to actually write in the book (why not, are you planning to sell it?), get a separate training log or make up your own. My guarantee is that by the end of the book the question won't be whether you're a walker. It will simply be, "What type of walker am I?" Daily foot-commuter or family hike organizer? After dinner ambler, or early morning jock? Avid mountain scrambler or tenacious 10K competitor? Unflagging marathoner or diligent neighborhood fitness walker? There is no right answer. But having experienced the variety of the one-year program, you'll know what's right for you.

We've also updated this edition with some of the most recent research and data on the health impacts of physical activity, all of it adding to the certitude of walking's far-reaching benefits. We've added more detailed information on walking with a pedometer, on using Nordic walking poles, and of special interest to me, on creating more walkable communities. One thing has become clear in my travels of recent years—you can have the best intentions in the world to exercise, but if your community makes it costly, dangerous, or even just inconvenient to do so, it's not going to happen. And the research bears this out—no sidewalks and sprawling community design means less walking. Meanwhile, you may not be planning to be active, but if your community makes it safe, convenient, cheap, and appealing—wide safe sidewalks, a corner store down the street and elementary school around the corner—then it's likely to happen without you even realizing it. Your activity may come from a walk to the bus stop instead of around a track, but with the right kind of community, it can and will happen. It also means you're more likely to be there when the kids are ready to jump off the bridge.

So please read and enjoy, but most of all, do more walking.

Part I

For the Health of It: Building a Daily Habit

Those who are now dodging the cemeteries will discover the vibrating forces of life easily within their reach. Many who are balancing themselves on the edge of the grave can find health and strength for many years of happiness through this simple prescription: Walk!

BERNARR McFADDEN
The Walking Cure, 1925

If we were meant to walk, we'd stand upright and have two legs and opposable thumbs.

MARK FENTON

1

Don't I Already Know How to Do This?

Trust walking

You must trust walking. That's the single most important thought I can give you. Believe that walking can and will make a difference in your life. I promise that even if you start with baby steps—even if your first walk is no more than 10 minutes long—regular daily walking will improve your health. Know that even if you have 30, 60, or 100 pounds to lose, thousands of people before you have done it successfully through diligent walking. Accept that even if you're an accomplished athlete who has taught aerobics classes or run marathons, vigorous walking can give you the same total energetic high and cardiovascular fitness as any other single activity, with far less damage to your body. And no matter what type of walker you become, know that it will give you self-confidence, balance, and even emotional calm in your life. Trust walking.

These days we are bombarded by the temptations of fads and quick fixes, empty weight-loss promises and dueling celebrity fitness experts. It's pretty easy to be confused about healthy living. Should you believe in meditation and herbs, reflexology and retreats, hormonal supplements and miracle drugs? Are any right for you? Will they make you healthier? One thing that I know will make you healthier—will absolutely reduce your risk of disease and an early death—is a brisk daily walk. Trust walking.

As I write this, high-protein, low-carbohydrate diets are all the rage. Should you cut out fat or layer it on with your breakfast bacon? Should you make whole-grain bread a staple or throw it out for the birds? Here's the answer: Let the diet "experts" argue and start burning calories with a vigorous daily walk. Eat smart every day. And trust walking.

With exercise, there's always a choice. You can bounce in aerobics class, punch and kick in tae bo, climb to nowhere on the Stairmaster, or run until your knees can take no more. Or you can head out for a vigorous walk and glide smoothly along the ground, feeling your legs driving, your arms pumping, and your heart working. Explore neighborhoods, climb hills, follow rivers, circle tracks, and at the end of it feel spent, but never beaten. Look forward to it again tomorrow. Trust walking.

And one more thing. We live in a world where we fear that our streets are unsafe. We now spend more time in automobiles than ever before. Traffic congestion and pollution threaten our sanity and our lungs. Neighborhood stores and schools are driven past, not walked to, and neighbors barely know one another by name. We live in communities that could stand to have a lot more people out walking a lot more of the time. You should be one of these pioneers. Walking is not only better for your spirit, mood, and body, it's better for your whole community. Trust walking.

The fact is, we do stand upright and have two legs and opposable thumbs. Our bodies are perfectly evolved for walking. That's why I'm not going to teach you how to walk. I'll teach you how to make walking a part of your life. You'll never forget it. You'll never stop doing it. You will trust walking.

QUIZ I
Kick Off Your Walking

In order to start your walking program at the right level, take the following quiz. It has three simple questions—just pick the best answer for you.

1. **How active is your average day?**
   a) Low key. Unless you count walking to the car, mailbox, fridge, or around the store, I'm either snoozing, sitting, or standing still.
   b) In gear. I'm often walking around at work, dashing up and down the stairs, or chasing kids.
   c) Overdrive. I have a physically demanding job or lifestyle that really keeps me moving (think river rafting guide, FedEx delivery person, or spinning instructor).

2. **How much conscious exercise do you get in a week?**
   a) Not much. I rarely get breathing hard, let alone break a real sweat.
   b) I'm trying. At least three days a week I get breathing hard enough—for at least 10 minutes—that if I were to answer the phone, the caller might ask what I was up to.
   c) I'm a jock. At least three days a week I work up enough of a sustained sweat to soak a shirt and need a shower afterward.

3. **How fit are you right now? If you warm up and then walk 1 mile at a hard, but not painful, pace, it takes:**
   a) More than 19 minutes.
   b) 14 to 19 minutes.
   c) Less than 14 minutes.

Score 1 point for an (a), 2 points for a (b), and 3 for a (c).

FOUR-WEEK WARM-UP PROGRAM
Take a walk for the number of minutes shown each day.

	Sun.	Mon.	Tue.	Wed.	Thu.	Fri.	Sat.
Week 1	10	10	(off)	10	10	10	(off)
Week 2	10	10	10	10	(off)	10	10
Week 3	10	15	10	(off)	10	15	10
Week 4	15	10	15	(off)	10	20	10

If you scored:

- **3 or 4 points.** Start with the Four-Week Warm-Up Program (see the box on page 3) before launching into the walking program. If the main program still feels too challenging, don't hesitate to repeat weeks 3 and 4 of this warm-up until you feel comfortable taking a sustained 20-minute walk.

- **5 to 7 points.** Follow the main program in this book exactly—it's designed perfectly for you. Literally head out tomorrow and do day number 1, a comfortable 20-minute walk (the program begins on page 20). Or if you want to begin on a Sunday, since that's how the program is shown, then take daily 15-minute walks between now and next Sunday. (Don't just sit around until then—get out and stroll.)

- **8 or 9 points.** You already have a fairly sound base level of fitness. You should read through weeks 17 to 24 of the program, beginning on page 79. If it looks reasonable and you feel you could do the workouts comfortably, start on week 17, with an easy 60-minute walk. If this feels like too much or you'd like to start more gradually, try beginning at week 9 (page 46). On the other hand, if you're already such an accomplished athlete that you don't even feel challenged, consider jumping right into the fitness segment of the program in week 33 (page 145).

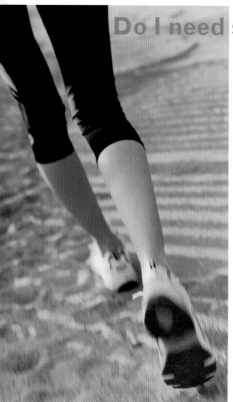

Do I need special shoes?

Later I'll talk about gearing up for walking. There's one piece of gear worth investing in even as a novice, however—a good pair of walking shoes. It's not worth messing around with cheap or old athletic shoes. (In any athletic shoe more than six months old, chances are that the cushioning doesn't have much life left—even if the shoe still looks fine.) I've seen too many people bail out of exercise programs because their feet hurt. That said, the $50 to $75 you're going to have to fork over for decent footwear shouldn't keep you from getting started—that's a lame reason to live with an elevated risk of a heart attack.

You have two choices for footwear—either athletic shoes or a pair of light hiking shoes, sometimes called rugged walking shoes. For sidewalks and roads, athletic shoes are ideal and tend to be lighter. In inclement weather or if you'll be venturing onto trails, you should probably go with a light hiking shoe.

Look first for shoes that are identified as walking shoes. Running shoes are a second choice; cross-trainers are third.

Specifically, look for the following:

- A shoe that bends easily through the ball of the foot but is fairly firm and won't bend easily through the arch.

- A low heel. Don't pick a running shoe with big, thick cushioning in the heel. The extra material in the heel tends to force your toes to slap down too quickly and can lead to shin discomfort as you walk.

- Stay away from high-tops (unless they're designed as walking or hiking shoes), because they can irritate your Achilles tendons. Also avoid shoes with extra layers and support straps. (These factors generally make basketball and aerobics shoes poor choices.)

The same criteria hold true for a light hiking shoe, keeping in mind that to offer more protection from rocks on the trail, the shoe won't be as flexible through the ball of the foot. It should also give you more lateral support (and perhaps a higher ankle) to protect against rolling your ankle.

Whatever else you do, be sure the shoes you walk in fit well and are among your most comfortable. That means the heel doesn't slip when you take a step, your toes never touch the end of the shoe, and there's no pinching or binding around the widest part of your foot, especially when you roll off your toes at the end of a step. There's no reason to be stopped by a blister before you've even started.

Walk Talk: Do I really have to visit the doctor before starting to exercise?

Many exercise programs say you should talk to your doctor before starting. They often have a very specific disclaimer—something like, "If you're very overweight or have any health conditions or are pregnant, or you're a man over 40 or a woman over 50, you should see the doctor before starting an exercise program."

Why the disclaimer? Is the jury still out on whether exercise is even safe? Certainly not. It's probably more reflective of how out of shape we've become as a society. People in the groups mentioned are at greater risk for complications if they suddenly take up vigorous physical activity. But frankly, it's a good idea for everyone to talk to a doctor before starting regular exercise. Your doctor knows your history and any special concerns you might have.

Keep in mind, however, that if your doctor isn't supportive of you becoming more active, it's time to get a new doctor. The majority of the medical community—from the surgeon general on down—agrees that regular physical activity is extremely important to long-term health. So give the doctor a call—she'll probably tell you to head out for a walk right now!

Anatomy of your first walk

Let's say you're ready to start with a 20-minute walk. You've got on some comfortable clothes and good walking shoes. Now what happens?

Focus on your walking time

Besides decent shoes and comfortable clothes, the only other equipment you might want for your walk is a watch. Head out the door, walk for 10 minutes in any direction, then turn around and come back. It's good to get in the habit of letting the clock—not the distance you've walked—measure your progress. That's because outdoor conditions and how you feel can vary a lot from day to day. A 15-block walk that seemed like a piece of cake on a cool spring morning could be tough at noon during the heat of summer. So initially it's better to target a time for your walks rather than a specific distance.

Of course, walking out and back on the same course can get boring fast. Also, the difference between a 15- and a 17-minute walk is pretty inconsequential. So use your first week or so of walking to figure out about how far you can go in various times. Find some 15-, 20-, and 30-minute loops; later, you can combine these to take even longer walks. Just be sure not to get hung up about covering a specific distance in a specific amount of time—you can focus on this later.

Go slow-fast-slow

Here are three simple tips for your first few walking workouts:

1. Start at your most comfortable pace. Spend the first three to five minutes letting your body get used to the idea of some sustained activity.
2. Next, pick it up and walk with purpose. This means that after warming up, you shouldn't stroll along as if you were window-shopping. Instead, walk as if it's a 10-minute walk to the office, and you've got a meeting starting promptly in 15 minutes.
3. Finish up at an easy pace again. The last few minutes should be comfortable, to allow your body to gradually cool down.

The anatomy of your walk forms a bell curve or upside-down letter *U*. Your effort starts low, rises up during the bulk of the walk, and drops down to finish. There are several reasons for this approach.

The easy start allows your body to warm up and your heart rate to rise and become prepared for an elevated level of activity. The temperature of your muscles and joints literally increases, making them more flexible and less prone to injury. Also, capillaries in your muscles dilate so that more blood can flow and more oxygen can be delivered to your working muscles.

Gradually cooling down the body can reduce the risk of your muscles tightening or cramping with an abrupt stop. It also gives your body time to bring some of the blood that was out at your extremities—supplying your muscles with oxygen—back to your core. This reduces the chance of light-headedness that might come with a sudden stop.

Five walking warm-up moves

The more intense the exercise you intend to do, the more you benefit from warm-up exercises. Keep in mind that gradually increasing blood flow and slowly increasing your muscle and joint temperature can improve your comfort and walking performance, and reduce the risk of injury during any walk. You'll feel better and walk better.

I recommend the following five simple moves before any brisk walk, because they target the muscles that do much of the work in walking. All are done standing up, and if you spend 30 seconds on each, the whole routine takes less than three minutes. (Rest one hand on something for balance when needed.)

1. Ankle circles. Stand on one foot and lift the other off the ground. Slowly flex that ankle through its full range of motion, making circles with the toes. Do 6 to 8 in each direction, then switch feet and repeat.

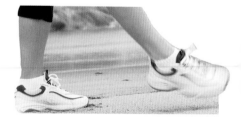

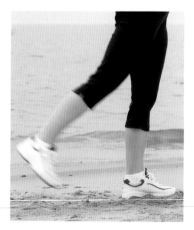

2. Leg swings. Stand on one leg and swing the other loosely from the hip, front to back. It should be a relaxed, unforced motion like the swinging of a pendulum, and your foot should swing no higher than a foot or so off the ground. Do 15 to 20 swings on each leg.

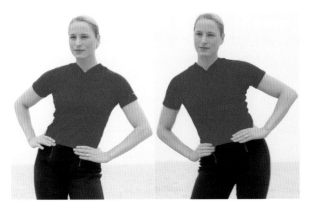

3. Pelvic loops. Put your hands on your hips with your knees gently bent and feet shoulder-width apart. Keep your body upright and make 10 slow, continuous circles with your hips, pushing them gently forward, to the left, back, and to the right. Then reverse directions and repeat.

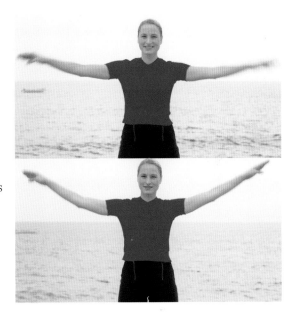

4. Arm circles. Hold both arms straight out to your sides, making yourself into the letter T. Make 10 to 12 slow backward circles with your hands, starting small and finishing with large circles, using your entire arm. Shake your arms out, then repeat with 10 to 12 forward circles.

5. Hula-hoop jumps. Begin hopping in place on both feet. Keep your head and shoulders facing forward, and twist your feet and lower body left, then right, back and forth, on successive hops, 20 times.

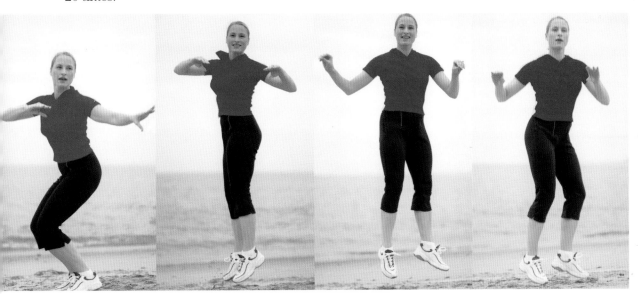

Walk Talk: What should I do to be safe while walking?

Most safety tips are pure common sense, but it's worth reminding yourself of them anyway, just in case.

- Always walk on a sidewalk when one is available, or on the left side of the street facing traffic. It's critical that you be able to see cars coming toward you.
- Know where you are and where you're going.
- Carry identification and perhaps a cell phone.
- Be aware that personal stereo headsets can make you less aware of your surroundings, of bicyclists or traffic, or of an approach by a stranger. Certainly never wear one in an unfamiliar area.
- If you're approached by a threatening dog, remain calm and try not to show fear. Say "no" and "go home" in a low, firm voice, but don't threaten the dog. Back away slowly if necessary. Of course, if it should attack, scream for help and fight back with all your might and any weapons you can grab—on two occasions I've avoided further problems with luck and a well-timed (and adrenaline-boosted) punch across the nose of charging dogs. In any case, for the benefit of the animal, notify the police or an animal control officer.
- Make yourself visible when walking in the dark, and especially at dawn and dusk, when visibility is deceptively poor. For best results:
  - Wear retro-reflective materials, not just light colors. Retro-reflectives (3M Scotchlite may be the best known) bounce light back toward its source, making them highly visible in car lights. Wear shoes and apparel with reflective fabric, logos, and trim, or wear a reflective vest.
  - Get 360-degree coverage. Cars come from the sides and front, too, so have reflective material all the way around, not just on your back.
  - Put reflective material on your moving parts. A bright spot on your wrist or ankle makes you look more like a person and less like a lane marker. (Think of the reflectors you've seen on bicycle pedals.)
  - Carry a flashlight. A small, high-quality light is easy to carry but throws enough light to be visible from a great distance.

Why Walking Must Be the Answer

George Carlin and the Surgeon General

Back in 1987, soon after *WALKING* Magazine was launched, comedian George Carlin took a playful swipe at the notion, I believe during a *Tonight Show* appearance. "*WALKING* Magazine? There's a *WALKING* Magazine?" he guffawed. "What's next, *Breathing* magazine?" Bada-bum. And in a sense, Carlin had it right. We know how to walk—what else is there to say about it?

On the other hand, he had it woefully wrong. Walking is one of our most natural and fundamental physical activities. Natural because our bodies have evolved to do it easily, efficiently, and comfortably. Fundamental because it's at the root of how we move around every day. Sure, we can run, jump, crawl, hop, even slither; some folks are pretty good swimmers. But most of us, when we're moving around under our own power, are walking.

Here's the problem: Most people aren't doing nearly enough walking. Or any other exercise, for that matter. In 1996 the surgeon general of the United States released a *Report on Physical Activity and Health*. It took a comprehensive look at all the research on physical activity and why it's good for us. The whole report boils down to two really critical findings, in my opinion:

- **Everyone should get at least 30 minutes of physical activity a day, most days of the week, to avoid an increased risk of many chronic diseases and an early death.**
- **Only about 25 percent of Americans actually get that daily 30-minutes through leisure time physical activity.**

This is a bit of classic good news and bad news. Good news because a daily 30-minute goal seems entirely reasonable. After all, the statement doesn't say you have to run 10 miles a day and do 200 push-ups. The report says a brisk 30-minute walk will do the trick just fine. But the fact that only one in four Americans makes time for that much exercise is quite bad news.

Even worse is the fact that when the report came out in 1996, the Centers for Disease Control estimated about 25 percent of Americans were essentially sedentary, getting no leisure-time physical activity at all. In a more recent survey the proportion of sedentary Americans approached 30 percent. So not only do many Americans fall short—some of us way short—of the surgeon general's recommendation, but the situation seems to be getting worse as well.

Americans may not need to learn *how* to walk, but we sure do need to learn how to walk *more*.

One more point. If you're not exercising at all, and certainly if you don't hit the 30-minute-per-day goal, don't waste a lot of energy feeling guilty. First of all, you're in the majority. Second, you sincerely want to make a change, and you have a blueprint for success right in your hands. The first 16 weeks of this walking program are designed specifically to help you create a complete and balanced lifestyle that includes walking and complementary activities. They ask only a moderate amount of time and will provide all of the benefits promised in the surgeon general's report.

What is walking good for?

Here's the quick answer: your heart, lungs, blood, muscles, bones and joints, brain, gastrointestinal tract, immune system, perhaps even eyes and ears, and most definitely mood and spirit. You can take my word for all this, or read a bit more below about the most well-researched and important benefits of daily walking.

Heart health

Cardiovascular disease is the number one killer of both men and women in the United States, and it has been for some time. The American Heart Association has for years cautioned against factors risky for our hearts, including smoking, a fat-laden diet, and stressful living. In 1992 it added another factor to this list, as dangerous as any other: physical inactivity. Studies consistently show that if you're sedentary, your risk of heart disease is substantially increased. They also show that just a little bit of walking can provide a lot of protection. Just 2 miles of walking a day, for example, has been shown to decrease heart disease risk by 30 to 40 percent.

The heart is a muscle, and it gets stronger with exercise just like any other muscle. A stronger heart is able to pump more blood more forcefully on every beat, and even actually end up taking fewer beats overall. The result: a muscle that's more likely to keep working well, and for a longer time.

Preventing osteoporosis

Osteoporosis is a great concern for aging adults, especially women over 40. Studies show that weight-bearing exercise is very important in staving off this dangerous reduction in bone density that seems to come naturally with age. Walking, combined with moderate strength training, is a

Walk Talk: Is it really true that walkers can get just as fit as runners, but are less likely to get hurt?

One of the most compelling studies I've been involved in was a 28-week research program focusing on walkers and runners at the University of Colorado. Two separate groups of women were sent to either walk or run 40 minutes a day, four days a week, at a moderately vigorous level. The participants were given technique instruction, were monitored by graduate students, and even learned how to check their heart rates and wear heart-rate monitors (to ensure that both walkers and joggers were giving the same effort).

Our hypothesis was simply that the walkers—even though they were walking very briskly—were less likely to be injured than the runners. We expected this because walkers only strike the ground with one to one and a half times their body weight, even at high speeds, while runners hit with three or more times their body weight on each stride. But the results were even more dramatic than we'd expected.

Both groups saw essentially the same improvements in aerobic fitness (as measured by before-and-after tread-mill tests). But the walkers suffered vastly fewer injuries, missing only a day and a half, on average, to injury. The runners, on the other hand, missed an average of about 11 days due to injuries, and in general their injuries were much more severe. Two women suffered stress fractures; another even required surgery!

Certainly not everyone who jogs gets injured; nor is everybody ready to work out as hard as the women in this study right away. But it sure is nice to know that even as you improve in fitness and pick up your walking pace, it's still going to be much easier on your bones and joints than running. You'll get just as fit as your jogging neighbor who's out literally pounding the pavement and his body, but with a lot less chance of getting hurt.

very good choice for maintaining bone density, and it's also a low-impact activity—which means the risk of acute injuries such as stress fractures is low. So walking is good for your bones in more ways than one: It stimulates them to stay strong, but it isn't likely to damage them in the process.

That said, don't presume that walking is sufficient protection against osteoporosis. A balanced diet with plenty of calcium is important, and it's clear that resistance training is very beneficial, particularly to the bones and joints of the upper body that see very little resistance during walking. (A progression of resistance-training programs—from novice to challenging—is included in the book.)

Managing diabetes

Diabetes is the inability to normally regulate and utilize glucose—the form of sugar in the bloodstream that your body uses for energy. Type II diabetes—formerly called adult-onset diabetes—is often associated with adult weight gain, and it can lead to severe complications, including heart disease, stroke, blindness, impaired circulation in the extremities, and eventually even amputations. And because it's now being seen in children, it is only referenced by its clinical name, Type II.

A major study, the Diabetes Prevention Program, proves the value of physical activity in managing Type II diabetes. The study compared conventional preventive counseling and diabetes medication with an intensive lifestyle change program in a population of people at risk for developing Type II diabetes (all had elevated fasting glucose levels but were not yet diabetic). The lifestyle change included an improved diet and walking at least 30 minutes a day, five days a week. Although those receiving medication saw a 31 percent reduction in risk of developing full-blown Type II, the real winners were the ones with improved diet and exercise habits; they experienced a 58 percent reduction in risk!

Although this 58-year-old hairdresser from Boston exudes energy, this wasn't always the case. "I hated exercise. Absolutely hated it," says Carol, remembering what life was like before she discovered walking. Having struggled with roller-coaster weight, back problems, and progressively worsening health in adulthood, it took no less than a physical collapse in 1991 for her to realize the extent of what was happening to her body. "One day at work I just fell off my feet, I was so exhausted. When the bloodwork came back we realized I was severely diabetic—my glucose was 825 milligrams per deciliter—and I'd never known it." With her metabolism so totally out of whack, the nurses were amazed that Carol had even gotten to the hospital under her own power. She eventually required two high-dosage insulin shots a day.

The Turning Point

Getting the exercise the doctor recommended was a struggle. "I'd tried all the fads, all the crash diets, all the quickie programs. I had thrown away a lot of money on health club memberships. I'd go twice a week for a while, then once, and then it would be over." In 1998 she took a three-month membership at the Athletic Center at nearby Roxbury Community College, largely because the track had a seniors exercise program based on walking. "With my back and my weight, walking seemed like the only thing that might work."

A Week in Her Life

Carol's trick is to cram lots of physical activity into the days when she has time for it, and to just make do when she's busy with her two jobs. She always attends a Monday and Wednesday exercise class, and a Friday class whenever time permits. Classes begin at 10 A.M., though many women arrive an hour earlier to start warm-ups—and to visit. "It helps to have an indoor place to walk. But most important is the camaraderie of the group. You get involved in each other's lives, you check up on each other. Before you know it, your miles are done."

Walks are followed by weight lifting and stretching. "Some days we'll dance, or do something else, too." For example, she's added a one-hour tennis class once a week.

On Tuesday and Thursday she strives for an informal walk by herself. Because her weekends are dominated by work, Carol piles most of her exercise into her three full mornings at the Athletic Center.

Her Biggest Accomplishment

It's as simple as this: Carol no longer needs insulin shots at all, a reversal that has drastically changed her life. "It's just so clear to me that the combination of a healthy diet and exercise is the key to keeping it under control. Plus you feel much better and have so much more energy."

Her Key to Success

Getting together with a group of people with a common goal. "We all came for different reasons—encouraged by a doctor, a desire to lose weight, whatever—but once we got involved, we realized there were so many reasons to show up every day. And you look forward to going, if for nothing else than to be with the others."

What's Next?

Carol wants to keep slowly and permanently lowering her weight and improving her metabolism. "My doctor is very proud of my gradual progress—just 10 or 15 pounds so far, nothing sudden or crazy—because he knows I can keep it off. He just wants me to keep doing what I'm doing."

Weighty matters

National research studies now estimate that more than 60 percent of Americans are overweight, and nearly one in three is medically obese. Fortunately, that research also gives a clear picture of what it takes to lose weight or maintain your weight loss and it was embodied nicely in the 2005 US Department of Agriculture (USDA) dietary recommendations. Though notable for its update of the food guide pyramid (see page 74), the USDA devoted an entire chapter of this document to physical activity, and it referenced among other sources compelling evidence coming out of the National Weight Control Registry (NWCR).

That study focuses on people who've lost significant weight and kept it off for two years or more, and it confirms the need to eat a moderate balanced diet and be physically active every day. But a surprise to some, says Dr. Jim Hill, a lead researcher at the University of Colorado on the NWCR, is the fact that one of the best predictors of success in weight loss, distinguishing successful long-term losers from those who lose but then regain weight, is daily physical activity. The most successful losers regularly accumulate 60 to as many as 90 minutes of activity a day. Note that for many it's not structured or even intense exercise, but rather accumulated activity throughout the day, such as walking to and from work. The simple point is that to maintain a healthy weight, physical activity must be part of your lifestyle.

Cancer count

In 1996, when the surgeon general's report on physical activity and health was published, the report suggested that the risk of colon cancer would be reduced among physically active adults. But at the time the authors were hesitant to make any greater claims. What a difference a decade makes. In the interim numerous studies have shown that physically active adults are at reduced risk for cancer in general, and according to the American Cancer Society, including regular physical activity in your day is as important as quitting smoking and eating a healthy diet in reducing your cancer risk.

Perhaps most compelling is the growing preponderance of evidence suggesting that physically active women are at reduced risk for breast cancer. Even more striking, a 2005 study in the *Journal of the American Medical Association* found that among women diagnosed with the disease, those walking three to five hours a week at an average pace are at reduced risk for death compared to sedentary women. So being physically active may help you not just prevent but even *fight* disease.

Emotional well-being

Of all the benefits of exercise, this one stands above all others. I've talked to people who have walked off 100 pounds or more, or have walked away from diabetes or high blood pressure. But the first thing they mention is how much better they feel about themselves.

Researchers have coined the phrase *health-related quality of life*, and they use it to measure the emotional benefits of exercise. Walkers use plain English to declare the joys of reduced stress, improved mood, growing self-confidence, and a sense of empowerment. Many regular walkers feel that they've taken control of their lives, and now the possibilities are limitless. Perhaps they'll lose more weight, or just maintain a healthy weight. But they believe they'll never put weight on again if they don't want to. Perhaps they'll remain neighborhood fitness walkers, or maybe they'll explore hiking or walking in road races or other sports. The important thing is that they believe in themselves as physical, capable beings.

Ditch the scale

To really be sure your walking is working, you need concrete measures of progress. Even if you're coming to this program with weight loss as a primary goal, however, I want you to know that the bathroom scale is not the best measure of your success. That's because even short-term fad diets can help you lose weight fast. For success over the long term, you need to permanently change your body, your metabolism, and, of course, your attitude. Unlike knocking off a few quick pounds, this will take time. The good news is that it's permanent, as long as you maintain your new way of life.

There are four concrete measures of your progress that will tell you more about your chances for a long and healthy life than the bathroom scale ever will. Together they comprise your metabolic fitness. They are blood pressure, cholesterol level, blood glucose level, and body mass index.

When you visit the doctor for a quick exam before starting your walking program, ask to get initial readings on these four indicators. Then come back for an update in 6 and in 12 months. Don't get frustrated if some of your readings are marginal or even high; it's better to know about these things and talk with your doctor about possible treatments. You're also taking a critical step toward improving them by starting this walking program!

Record your metabolic fitness

Write down all the readings from this section at the beginning of the walking program log (page 20). The program will then remind you to measure them again in 6 and 12 months.

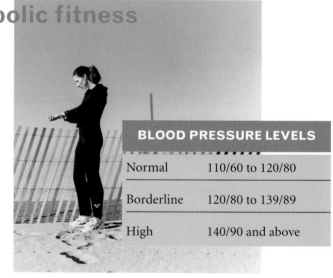

BLOOD PRESSURE LEVELS	
Normal	110/60 to 120/80
Borderline	120/80 to 139/89
High	140/90 and above

1. **Blood pressure.** You know that high blood pressure is a risk factor for heart disease, but do you know what your blood pressure is? You should. It's made up of two numbers, *systolic* and *diastolic* pressure (measured in millimeters of mercury), stated as one over the other. The first number essentially measures the pressure when the heart is beating; the second is the pressure during the recovery time between beats.

2. **Cholesterol levels.** Triglycerides are fatty substances in the blood, and it's well known that high levels can contribute to clogged arteries and cardiovascular problems. Check your

CHOLESTEROL LEVELS

	Total	LDL	HDL
Healthy	less than 200 mg/dl	less than 130 mg/dl	Men: over 40 mg/dl; Women: over 50 mg/dl
Marginal	200 to 239 mg/dl	130 to 159 mg/dl	
At Risk	more than 239 mg/dl	more than 159 mg/dl	Men: under 40 mg/dl; Women: under 50 mg/dl

levels of total triglycerides, LDL (so-called bad cholesterol), and HDL (the good stuff: higher levels of HDL are associated with improved heart health because the substance may help clear blood vessels). Your measurements will be expressed in milligrams of fat per deciliter of blood (mg/dl), and remember that higher levels of HDL are a good thing.

3. **Blood glucose levels.** Diabetes is an excess of glucose (a type of sugar) in your blood because of a metabolic inability to process it properly. Approximately 20.8 million Americans are estimated to suffer from diabetes, with roughly 6.2 million unaware that they even have the disease, so it's well worth having your blood glucose levels checked—and all the more so because regular exercise is likely to have a positive impact on your readings. Results of a fasting plasma glucose test (FPGT) will be stated in milligrams of glucose per deciliter of blood (mg/dl).

BLOOD GLUCOSE LEVELS	
Normal	60 to 100 mg/dl
Pre-diabetic	110 to 125 mg/dl
Diabetic	more than 125 mg/dl

4. **Body mass index,** or BMI, is a much better way to look at your weight than simply measuring it on the bathroom scale. BMI takes into account both your height and weight, and recognizes the fact that taller people are likely to be heavier. To calculate your BMI, follow these steps:

- Weigh yourself for three days in a row, first thing in the morning after you go to the bathroom. Add these together and divide by three to get an average. (Then put the scale away—it's not your focus.)
- Determine your height, in bare or stocking feet, in inches.
- Multiply your weight in pounds by 703.
- Divide that result by your height in inches; divide that result again by your height in inches. The result is your BMI, expressed in kilograms per square meter (kg/m^2).

For example: Gertrude is 5 foot 3 (63 inches) and weighs 143 pounds. She multiplies 143 by 703 ($143 \times 703 = 100{,}529$). Then she divides by 63 ($100{,}529 \div 63 = 1{,}596$) and by 63 again ($1{,}596 \div 63 = 25.3$). Her BMI is 25.3.

Keep in mind that the BMI doesn't take into account body composition—whether you're made up of more fat or muscle. A pro football player might be very muscular and therefore heavy for his height—with a BMI of more than 28—but still fairly healthy. On the other hand, if you lack muscle tone but are only slightly overweight according to the BMI (like Gertrude), you should still be concerned with building muscle and losing fat.

BMI	
Normal	less than 25 kg/m^2
Overweight	25 to 30 kg/m^2
Obese	more than 30 kg/m^2

5. Body measurements (optional). There's nothing wrong with the fact that some of your motivation for exercising may be that it will help you feel better about your body. Not just physically better—less random soreness and stiffness when you get up in the morning, more confidence that you can do things—but emotionally better. This isn't something that happens overnight, but over the course of this book and one-year plan you'll definitely see changes that will make you smile. So take the following measurements now with a cloth tape measure:

- Thigh. Measure around the thickest part of the upper leg.
- Upper arm. Measure around the thickest part.
- Waist-to-hip ratio. Measure your waist at the top of your hip bones, and your hips at the widest point. Divide waist by hip. For example, if your waist is 32 inches and your hips are 38, then the ratio would be 32 ÷ 38, or 0.84.

Note that a smaller waist-to-hip ratio tends to be healthier, but in general you're measuring so that you can watch for change over time. Your ratio should drop as you firm up and trim down. Your upper-arm and thigh measurements are also likely to drop if you're overweight, though if you're thin but not in great shape you might not see them change much. You will, however, notice that your arms and thighs get toned as you get stronger and build a bit of muscle.

Get moving every day

If this is your first serious attempt at regular exercise, or if you've tried before and failed, you may have two things in common with a lot of Americans. One, you know you're supposed to exercise because it's good for you. And two, you figure it's going to take a lot of time, hard work, and maybe even suffering for you to really see any benefits. Here's the problem: You're only half right.

You're right about the myriad benefits of physical activity—but you're wrong about how hard it is to receive them. As I've said, even a modest amount of daily movement can offer great health benefits. It won't get you in shape for the Olympic team, of course, but you're not trying to go to the Olympics. That comes later. For now, lowering your cholesterol a few points, shedding a few pounds, dropping away from borderline high blood pressure, and feeling a little better would be great. Think of yourself as starting at the base level of an activity pyramid that consists of three levels: health and well-being, weight loss, and total fitness.

Begin at the base

The base of the activity pyramid is the foundation on which an active, healthy lifestyle is built. It boils down to this: Walking purposefully for 30 minutes per day, combined with simple, regular stretching, is enough to improve your health and lower your risk of chronic disease. The term *purposefully* means you're walking as if trying to get somewhere, not just sauntering along smelling the flowers or window-shopping. You feel no urge to break into a run, but you're moving along smartly. For most people, this is in the 3- to 4-mile-per-hour range. If you're very heavy or haven't been active in years, your pace might be slower, but 3 miles per hour (about 20 minutes for a mile) is a good minimum target. In addition, flexibility work helps to maintain a healthy range of movement and avoid injuries in your muscles and joints. Once you've mastered the habits at the base of the pyramid, you can tackle more, but for starters focus on daily walking and regular stretching (see chapter 4 for proper stretching).

The Activity Pyramid

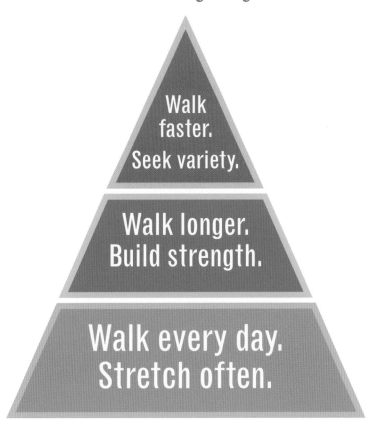

Walk
faster.
Seek variety.

Walk longer.
Build strength.

Walk every day.
Stretch often.

Start at the bottom: Walking purposefully for 30 minutes per day,
combined with simple, regular stretching, is enough to improve your
health and lower your risk of chronic disease.

Is 30 minutes a day enough?

I often find that people presume the base of the pyramid is for athletic losers; folks who lack the skill or talent for competitive sports, or can't handle anything more challenging. I'm happy to say I now have a pretty healthy perspective on this, perhaps thanks to two children. When I was competing on the U.S. National Racewalking Team, my life revolved around exercise; we often tackled 20-mile endurance walks or high-speed interval workouts at a faster-than-seven-minute-per-mile pace (about 8.5 miles per hour). In my current postcompetitive life with a son and daughter, however, I don't have the time or inclination for such things. I often settle for quick jaunts on foot to the store, paddling the kids in the kayak, or chasing (and I mean *chasing!*) them around a soccer field. I'm not throwing in the towel on exercise. I'm focusing on the base of the pyramid right now and finding more ways to get my 30 minutes per day. Meanwhile, my forays up the pyramid aren't necessarily traditional workouts, though they're still a lot of fun. But now it's probably more important than ever to my long-term health to make sure I get at least 30 minutes a day.

Why should you be at least at the base of the pyramid, even if you've been more active (or less) before? Because you simply can't put the health benefits of exercise in the bank. All the physiological benefits and reduced risks that come with exercise depend on a consistent, daily dose of activity. Stop walking every day and the protective effects wane. So the base of the pyramid is the minimum you want to strive for, and never fall below.

Walk Talk: My days are packed; I'm going nonstop. I'm sure that I get in 30 minutes of activity without even knowing it, right?

Not necessarily. Don't confuse being busy with being physically active. One hundred years ago, being busy probably meant working in a factory or doing chores on a farm. But many of the things that consume tons of time in modern life don't have a thing to do with being physically active. If you want to tally your active time in a day, check out the chart below for some reminders as to what counts and what doesn't. As a general rule, activities that require the substantial and frequent movement of your major muscle groups—legs, torso, arms, and shoulders—count toward your daily 30-minute goal. Anything less, even if it makes you tired, probably doesn't make you any healthier.

BUSY: Don't Count It Toward Physical Activity	ACTIVE: Count It Toward Your 30 Minutes
Driving to four different meetings at four different office buildings.	Walking to four different buildings (or to the bus or subway) to get to four meetings.
Changing a diaper, reading a book, feeding a three-year-old.	Playing tag, going for a walk, being Horsie for a three-year-old.
Answering 27 e-mails.	Taking the stairs seven flights up to talk to one real person.
Being caught in traffic.	Riding your bike instead of driving.
Organizing and paying bills.	Organizing, dusting, and vacuuming the living room. Fast.
Driving kids to soccer, band, and a friend's house.	Running drills and shagging balls at soccer practice.
Cutting up vegetables, making dinner.	Planting vegetables, weeding a garden.

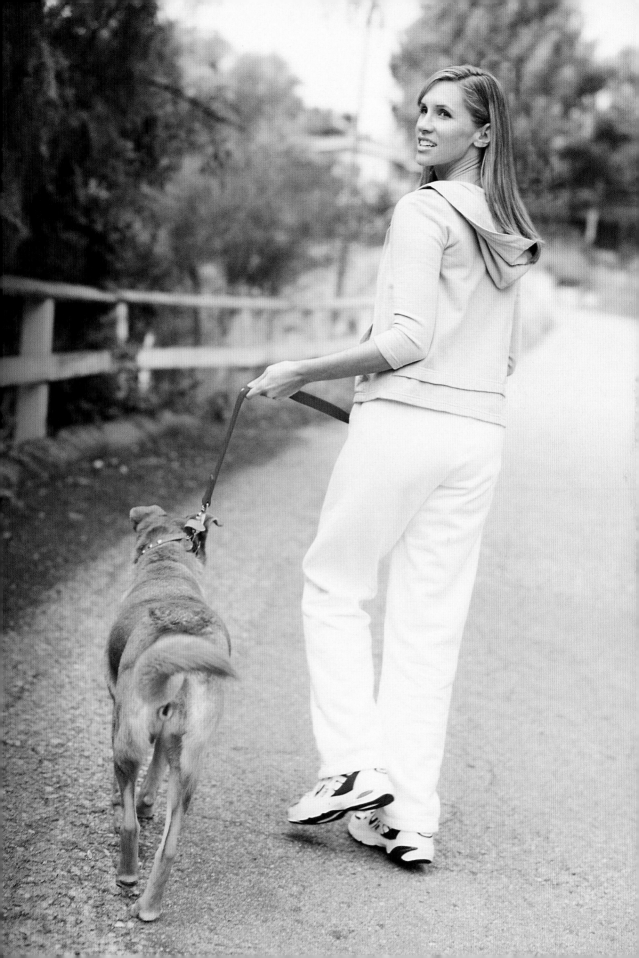

Make walking part of your life

This program recognizes that you're busy and have lots of priorities. Being active is one priority, and it has to fit into a realistic schedule. The following recommendations allow for lots of day-to-day variety. They encourage longer and shorter walks, faster and slower ones, and plenty of walks that you can sneak in during the day—say, as part of a commute to work, walking the kids to a friend's house, or walking with a colleague during your lunch hour. The point is, don't look at these schedules as workouts. Look at them as reminders to find active opportunities in your day.

The rules

1. **Walk or be active practically every day.** Every day, the number of minutes to walk is recommended. Even if you can walk only 5 or 10 minutes, however, remember that it's a lot better than doing nothing at all.
2. **Write it down.** At the very least put a check mark next to the walk if you achieved it that day or put a zero (0) if you did nothing. Estimate the mileage you walked if you feel you'd like to keep a running total (which I recommend).
3. **Rearrange at will.** The recommendations begin with 10- to 20-minute walks but eventually build up to an hour and longer. Swap days to fit your schedule. Take shorter walks on your busiest days. Take longer walks or do additional activities when you have more time. Don't feel bound to try to do the specific workouts on the days I recommend them; make the program fit *your* schedule.
4. **Spread out the longer days.** Try not to bunch the longest walks of the week on back-to-back days. Give your body some variety and time to rest.
5. **Listen to your body.** Take the "Kick Off Your Walking" quiz in chapter 1 to make sure you're starting at the right place. If you're feeling tired or sore from walking, back off a bit. If this isn't challenging enough, skip ahead a few weeks.
6. **Walk or be active practically every day.** It's a rule important enough to repeat. Break your walks into 10-minute chunks if need be, go early in the day or go late—but try to do some walking at least six days a week, and find ways to be more active every day.

RECORD YOUR METABOLIC FITNESS			
	Week 1	**Week 26**	**Week 52**
Blood Pressure			
Cholesterol Total/LDL			
Blood Glucose			
Body Mass Index			

	Date	Today's Activity Goal(s)	Total Minutes (or √)	Stretch? (√)	Comments, Other Activities? (vigorous chores, sports, other exercise, etc.)	Estimated Miles Walked
Sunday		15				
Monday		10				
Tuesday		15				
Wednesday		10				
Thursday		15				
Friday		off				
Saturday		20				

Miles this week: _____

Total miles for the year: _____

Log it every day

Get in the habit of looking at this log every day. In the "Total Minutes" column write down how many minutes you walked, or simply put a check if you did exactly the recommendation. Put in a 0 if you didn't walk—that's an important reminder (and powerful motivator) to get out and walk tomorrow!

You may also find tallying your total mileage inspiring—just jot down roughly how many miles you walk each day, then add them up for the week. Not sure how many miles your walks cover? Estimate 1 mile for every 20-minute walk; when you get faster, you can bump it up to 1 mile for every 15 minutes. (For convenience, estimate to the nearest 0.5 mile.)

Tip for the week. **Keep this book and a pen right next to your bed so you can fill it in every night before you go to sleep and plan your walk in the morning when you wake up.**

	Date	Today's Activity Goal(s)	Total Minutes (or √)	Stretch? (√)	Comments, Other Activities? (vigorous chores, sports, other exercise, etc.)	Estimated Miles Walked
Sunday		15				
Monday		15				
Tuesday		15				
Wednesday		10				
Thursday		15				
Friday		off				
Saturday		25				

Miles this week: _____

Total miles for the year: _____

Shoot for one day off a week—no more

Every week shows a day off on Friday, with no walking recommended. That's the perfect day to take a walk you missed earlier in the week, or to take Saturday's walk if you know you won't have time for it then, so you still get in six days of activity. But if you do all the walks as recommended, try doing something else on Friday: hop in a pool, go for a bike ride, toss the Frisbee with your kids, push the lawn mower, take a yoga class. Just because there's no walk scheduled doesn't mean you should be a slug. Just look for other ways to be active.

Tip for the week. **Feel free to substitute or count other aerobic activities toward your walking total occasionally. Just be sure it's an activity in which you move your major muscle groups fairly continuously (anything from digging in the garden to aerobics or swimming) for at least as long as the recommended walking time.**

	Date	Today's Activity Goal(s)	Total Minutes (or √)	Stretch? (√)	Comments, Other Activities? (vigorous chores, sports, other exercise, etc.)	Estimated Miles Walked
Sunday		15				
Monday		20				
Tuesday		15				
Wednesday		10				
Thursday		20				
Friday		off				
Saturday		25				

Miles this week: ———————

Total miles for the year: ———————

Start tallying your miles for the year

You'll be amazed at how inspiring it is to actually measure the total number of miles you walk. It won't seem like much now—probably just 5 miles a week or so—but they add up fast. At the end of each week, total all the miles you've walked and add it to your current total for the year. Then when you turn to the next page of the program, carry the figure forward and put it in the "Total miles for the year." In a few months you'll be downright impressed with yourself.

Tip for the week. **Try this game—flip ahead to weeks 26 and 52 and write down how many miles you estimate you will have totaled when you get to those weeks. Then no peeking until you get there!**

	Date	Today's Activity Goal(s)	Total Minutes (or √)	Stretch? (√)	Comments, Other Activities? (vigorous chores, sports, other exercise, etc.)	Estimated Miles Walked
Sunday		15				
Monday		20				
Tuesday		15				
Wednesday		10				
Thursday		25				
Friday		off				
Saturday		30				

Miles this week: _____

Total miles for the year: _____

Try using a pedometer during your walks

In the motivational tips in chapter 3, a lot of space is devoted to the idea of using a pedometer (or step counter) to help keep you moving and measure your progress. If you haven't tried one already and you're having trouble getting in your walks every day, it's time to give a pedometer a whirl. It's a modest investment, and I think you'll find one fun and easy to use. (See "Pedometers" in the resource list at the end of this book.)

Tip for the week. Put your pedometer on your hip as you head out the door to the post office, the corner store, or just around the block. Then don't think about timing your walk; just try to reach the number of steps equal to the recommended walk for the day. For starters, five minutes of walking equals about 600 steps (or 120 steps a minute).

Minutes	Steps to Shoot For
10	1,200
15	1,800
20	2,400
25	3,000
30	3,600
40	4,800

Date	Today's Activity Goal(s)	Total Minutes (or √)	Stretch? (√)	Comments, Other Activities? (vigorous chores, sports, other exercise, etc.)	Estimated Miles Walked
Sunday	15				
Monday	20				
Tuesday	20				
Wednesday	15				
Thursday	25				
Friday	off				
Saturday	30				

Miles this week: _____

Total miles for the year: _____

Add four minutes of stretching to your daily habit

In chapter 4 a simple three-move stretching routine is introduced. All the moves can be done standing up right after your walk, so wet ground or the lack of an exercise mat is no excuse to skip stretching. Even better, if you do each move just once, the routine can take as little as four minutes. Yet it can be an important part of maintaining your overall range of motion as well as muscle and joint health.

This week try doing that simple stand-up routine (found on page 42) after at least two or three of your walks. On the days you do stretch for a few minutes, check off under "Stretch?" in the log.

Tip for the week. Eventually your goal should be to stretch after every walk, but while you're building the habit, make sure you stretch at least after your three most vigorous efforts. That includes your longer outings, as well as faster walks or rambles on more hilly terrain.

	Date	Today's Activity Goal(s)	Total Minutes (or √)	Stretch? (√)	Comments, Other Activities? (vigorous chores, sports, other exercise, etc.)	Estimated Miles Walked
WEEK 6						
Sunday		15				
Monday		25				
Tuesday		15				
Wednesday		20				
Thursday		25				
Friday		off				
Saturday		35				

Miles this week: _____

Total miles for the year: _____

Wear your pedometer all day long

A terrific way to use a pedometer for motivation is to get in the habit of wearing it from the moment you get up in the morning until you go to bed at night. Then simply try to gradually increase the number of steps you take all day long. Many exercise experts feel that accumulating 10,000 steps over an entire day is similar to meeting the surgeon general's recommendation of adding 30 minutes of exercise walking a day, so this can be an eventual goal. Time to skip the elevator and start walking up the stairs! (For more pedometer ideas see page 34.)

Tip for the week. Measure how many steps you get in normal daily life by wearing your pedometer all day for several days *except* when you head out specifically for walks. Then, after you know your typical daily step level, try to reach that *plus* an amount equal to the daily walking recommendations (figuring 120 steps a minute). So if you find you typically take about 3,000 steps a day without consciously exercising, and the day's recommendation is 20 minutes (2,400 steps), your total goal for the day should be 5,400 steps.

	Date	Today's Activity Goal(s)	Total Minutes (or √)	Stretch? (√)	Comments, Other Activities? (vigorous chores, sports, other exercise, etc.)	Estimated Miles Walked
Sunday		15				
Monday		25				
Tuesday		15				
Wednesday		20				
Thursday		30				
Friday		off				
Saturday		35				

Miles this week: ———————

Total miles for the year: ———————

Don't fixate on time— focus on *daily* walking

The program varies from day to day to give you mental and physical variety, and to help you fit it into your weekly schedule. But you shouldn't be obsessed about hitting exactly the recommended time each day. If you're feeling good and walking farther now and then, that's terrific. The important thing is to follow the general trend of the program.

Tip for the week. These are the key habits you should be building.

- The length of your walks varies somewhat—you don't always walk the same loop and time.
- Overall you're gradually increasing the number of minutes you walk each week.
- You don't miss walking more than one day a week.
- You stretch for at least a few minutes after most of your walks.

Date	Today's Activity Goal(s)	Total Minutes (or √)	Stretch? (√)	Comments, Other Activities? (vigorous chores, sports, other exercise, etc.)	Estimated Miles Walked
Sunday	15				
Monday	25				
Tuesday	15				
Wednesday	20				
Thursday	30				
Friday	off				
Saturday	40				

Miles this week: _____

Total miles for the year: _____

How is your healthy habit progressing?

You've been walking for eight weeks already, and if you've followed the program exactly, you've walked 48 days. Look back at the log and count how many days you've checked off or exceeded the recommendation.

- **44 or more.** You're building a stupendous habit (averaging about six days a week).
- **36 to 43.** Solid performance—keep it up (averaging five days a week).
- **28 to 35.** You're walking more days than you don't (about four days a week), but you could do more.
- **20 to 27.** Try for just 10-minute walks on the days you're missing to begin improving.

Tips for the week. **If you've walked fewer than 20 days, it's time to renew your commitment to getting out the door. Recruit a partner, set a specific walking time, and keep at it. Also, get a pedometer and try to boost your daily step total by just 1,000 steps.**

3

Making It
Seem Easy

It's all about motivation

What should you do to make sure your 30 minutes of daily walking happens? Absolutely, positively whatever it takes. That's how important a daily walking habit really is. But you have to start with the realization that your personal motivation is the key to success. Bonnie Stein, a magnificent racewalking instructor in Florida, often asks her classes, "If I could pay you one hundred dollars a day to exercise for an hour, how many of you could find the time to do it?" Most people raise their hands. Stein then points out that exercise is simply a question of priorities. They *could* find the time to exercise right now. The $100 incentive would simply move exercise up on their priority lists.

Of course, the benefits of daily activity far surpass $100 per day, and at least intellectually you understand that it's a priority. This is why I believe the critical first step is creating the daily habit of getting out the door. Your focus at first shouldn't be on the speed or the duration of your walks, but simply on making them happen daily. In helping people to create a daily walking habit I have found four key elements are very helpful in assuring success.

Bite off *less* than you can chew

Dr. Russ Pate, an exercise physiologist at the University of South Carolina, once offered me this pearl of wisdom: "Pain is definitely not positively reinforcing." In other words, if something hurts, you probably won't do it again. This is precisely why initially you're much better off if you take on a little *less* walking than you can handle. Taking it easy at first ensures that you'll feel good at the end of each walk, not exhausted. This in turn increases the chance that you'll actually look forward to walking tomorrow, as opposed to dreading your next effort. It explains why the early

Mel Smagorinsky is a 69-year-old with the fitness of a 50-year-old (according to his doctor)—thanks to a walking habit that began long before it was cool. In fact, it was downright cold! A walking role model from my hometown of Brockport in western New York State, Mr. Smagorinsky bundled himself against a driven snow and strode purposefully to work while I struggled vainly to shovel the driveway. At the time I didn't see anything extraordinary about his effort—he was just a friend who walked to work at the local college *every single day*. But I suspect his habit abetted my assumption that it was perfectly normal to walk to school daily.

The Turning Point

Mel's fundamental approach: Walk when others would normally drive. Walking to work, the grocery store, and the post office have helped him maintain a lifelong commitment. But most critical has been his consistency through even the harshest winters of the upstate New York snow belt. How did he do it? "I learned how to outfit myself. I wore a heavy winter coat with hood and one of those Russian-style hats with the furry flaps. On the worst days I'd wear a mask that skiers use, and even ski goggles."

Wouldn't It Have Been Easier to Drive?

"In the bad winters we used to have, I could walk the mile and a half home faster than someone trying to drive. I'd watch the cars struggling up the hill on the ice, and I'd literally walk right by them." Has he ever not walked due to weather? "Not that I can recall."

A Week in His Life

When he was working, Mel walked to and from work daily plus up the stairs to his sixth-floor office. When he retired, he continued to have his *New York Times* delivered to the college just so he could walk

weeks of the program seem pretty modest. You can always walk longer than the recommendations. But in the beginning it's good to finish a walk feeling like you could do a bit more, not like you absolutely tested your limit.

Keep in mind that serious physical pain from walking is pretty unlikely, no matter how poor your fitness. Certainly you might get winded if you try charging up a hill, or feel some muscle soreness the next day if you try to go too far. But just as likely is mental pain—frustration at trying to carve 30 minutes out of your day or irritation at how out of shape you've let yourself become. So seriously consider my advice to start slowly. You'll avoid mental anguish as well as physical discomfort.

Take your time adding time

I have a fairly clear rule of thumb here: From one week to the next, never add more than 10 to 20 percent to the total number of minutes (or miles) you walk in a week. Don't worry—this rule is easier to adhere to than you think.

Let's say you walked for 15 minutes six out of seven days last week. That's a total of 90 minutes to pick it up. Now he intersperses a variety of activities into his week. A 30- to 40-minute walk is still his daily standard, but on many Tuesdays and Thursdays through the summer he replaces it with two hours of tennis; in winter he substitues a Nautilus strength-training program at the gym. He also tends to take Saturday off when family or social obligations call.

His Biggest Accomplishment

Nothing less than making walks a routine part of his day. His trip to work was primary, but Mel has made a point of running errands on foot, too. "If we needed milk, I'd forgo the car, carry a knapsack, and walk to the store. In retirement I'm even more conscious of going on foot." Once the kids moved out, he and his wife went down to one car because that's all they found they needed.

His Key to Success

"The key word is *commitment*. You have to decide that this is an important part of your life, and always find reasons to be out walking." And what about those upstate winters? "People would often offer a ride, but I'd rarely accept. I know myself and my routine, and I never wanted to give myself a reason or excuse to pass up a walk."

What's Next?

"Now that I'm older, I don't take on the same weather I might have when I was working." He sometimes hops on the treadmill, or even walks at a mall occasionally. Mel's always on the alert for new places to walk. "I saw a sign at the ice rink at the college: NO RUNNING AROUND THE RINK. I would have never thought of it—I didn't realize there was a nice continuous walkway up there. But it's like an invitation. Hey, it didn't say NO WALKING!"

of walking. Ten percent of that is 9 minutes; 20 percent of it is 18 minutes. So it's reasonable to add about 15 minutes of walking this week—somewhere between 9 and 18 minutes. However, I wouldn't recommend you add all 15 of those minutes to a single day. Instead, you might add 5 minutes to three of your daily walks. For example, you'd walk 15 minutes on three days and 20 minutes on three other days. To top it off, you could mix up the 15- and 20-minute days to give your body a little variety.

You'll see that I stick to this rule pretty carefully in the program in this book. I feel it's a useful way to keep yourself feeling comfortable, looking forward to more, and avoiding injury while also being sure that you're building toward improved fitness.

Don't let a stumble become a fall

I have a friend who was starting to exercise for the first time in a long time. I encouraged her to try a 90-day walking program I'd designed. It started with 10-minute daily walks and built up to 30 minutes per day. In the program I required her to walk only six days per week; on the seventh she could take a day off or do whatever she chose. She started off fine.

Then she had a really busy week at work, one of her kids got sick, and she missed a couple of days of walking. The next time we spoke she had bailed out of the program altogether. I was devastated and almost killed myself.

Well, no, I maintained my grip, but I was very unhappy that she'd quit. I told her to relax, not to worry about the missed days, and start again where she left off. I also offered the following tips:

- Be flexible about which day of the week you take off—make it your busiest day in any given week. It doesn't necessarily have to be the same day every week.

- Remember that something is always better than nothing. Even if you intended to walk 20 minutes, a 10-minute walk is still vastly better for you than doing nothing.

- Accept the fact that some weeks you'll miss more days than others. Don't sweat it.

- Even if you miss a bunch of days or even weeks, know that you're still better off starting again. Every step you've already taken means you'll be back to your previous level faster than the last time.

My friend mistakenly assumed that after the missed week, she had to start all over. Following our talk she was able to start up again guilt-free, this time more quickly, and she made real progress.

Keep it fun

Sure, this is entirely self-evident, but you'd be amazed at the number of people who seem to forget that making their exercise fun is a great path to success. Conversely, letting your walking be a chore is a sure path to failure. So do everything in your power to make your daily walks enjoyable.

I'm a firm believer that the simple act of getting outdoors, breathing fresh air, and seeing and experiencing my surroundings on foot is innately enjoyable. But don't hesitate to add to your pleasure: Walk with a friend, pick nice destinations or loops, take a dog you love, carry a picnic, train for a race, walk at sunrise or sunset. (For example, check out chapter 16 for information on walking events, from casual to competitive.) I'll offer thoughts on this throughout the book, but in short, do whatever you can to make your daily walk something you look forward to. In the end it's not how much healthier your heart is or how many pounds you lose, but your enjoyment of walking that will determine whether it becomes a permanent part of your life.

QUIZ II
Match Your Style
Everyone finds different ways to fit walking into their lives, and you'll have to discover what works best for you. I can help this process along by asking you to take a quick look at your lifestyle. Select the answers below that describe you best. Then, using your quiz results as a guide, look at the motivational tips that follow to find those best suited to your style.

1. **When you get out of the bed in the morning, what do you expect from your day?**
   a) I haven't a clue where I'll be eating lunch or when I'll have dinner. My day has to be flexible to respond to the demands and needs of children, work, family, and friends.
   b) I have a guess where I'll eat lunch and a fairly good idea of dinnertime. I usually have a few specific plans or priorities in the day, but plenty of free-form time, too.
   c) I know where I'll have lunch and exactly when dinner is planned. I keep a daily calendar and follow my intended schedule quite closely.

2. You have things you should drop off at four friends' homes today. How is it most likely to happen?

a) I'll get to each one whenever I think of it, maybe during lulls; hopefully I'll get to all of them today.

b) I'll try to adjust my plans a little to get to each one when I'm in the area; I'll get to them all before the day is over.

c) I'll build my schedule so that it fits optimally into the other things I'll be doing during the day, and I'll get to all of them by noon.

3. You're making dinner plans with close friends, and are picking a restaurant together. Will you:

a) Offer few opinions, and happily go wherever everyone else picks?

b) Offer several ideas and describe your choices glowingly, but willingly go with the majority?

c) Be very clear about your one or two picks, and try hard to convince people they're the best choices?

Score 1 point for an (a), 2 points for a (b), and 3 for a (c).

• **3 or 4 points.** Consider a *flexible* approach. You can plan on fewer formal workouts, and focus instead on accumulating your activity throughout the day.

Gear that might help: A simple but high-quality pedometer that counts your steps, and a simple calendar to act as a training log (like the one in this book). Wearing a pedometer several days of the week can give you a different look at your activity level. And scheduling walking into your calendar may help you hit your goal for the day.

• **5 to 7 points.** Follow a *balanced* approach. Focus on entertainment and keeping engaged, incorporating some tips from the flexible approach and some from the structured approach.

Gear that might help: A training log, an inexpensive athletic watch, and an inexpensive pedometer. You may want to time your formal workout walks and wear a pedometer for busier days to tally your total walking. Keep the log by your bed and take just a minute each night to jot down what you did that day.

• **8 or 9 points.** Follow a more *structured* approach to walking. Consider walking with groups, doing formal events, or going to a track somewhat regularly for timed and measured efforts.

Gear that might help: A quality digital athletic watch with stopwatch function, to time structured workouts. You might want to use a calendar to write in your planned workouts for the week ahead of time. Schedule the shorter walks on your busiest days, and check off your workouts when completed.

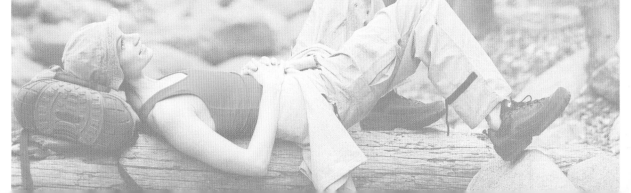

The tricks of the trade, from flexible to structured

The "Match Your Style" quiz gives you an informal look at your exercise personality. It's much too simple to be definitive, but I've found it's not a bad guide to helping people think about which motivational tricks will work for them. Below are some of the many devices you can use to motivate, inspire, and even trick yourself into your daily walks. They are listed roughly from those most suited to a flexible exercise lifestyle—people who need to be able to squeeze their walking in around other very unstructured activities—to those best for structured exercisers. So the lower your score on the quiz, the more you might like tips at the beginning of the list; the higher your score, the more you might prefer the tips at the end.

Count steps—using a pedometer

Pedometers are all the rage in exercise and weight-loss programs, but for many people they turn out to be more of a short-term novelty than an effective activity-promotion tool. For that reason I wrote the book *Pedometer Walking* with my friend and University of Tennessee exercise physiologist (and pedometer expert) David Bassett. In it we lay out a simple research-based approach that's likely to help even the least organized, most "unstructured" people add more activity to their days. We call it the "20 Percent Boost" program, and the idea is disarmingly simple.

When you first get a pedometer, don't try to increase your exercise or walking at all. Instead, wear the pedometer for one week and just live your normal daily life. Put the pedometer on when you first wake up in the morning—even on your pajamas—and keep it on all day until bedtime, except when you're submerged in water or naked (ouch). Place your pedometer on your waistband or belt, making sure that it's upright and not tilted front-to-back or side-to-side. It should be in front of your hip, in line with one knee. And this is important: Don't think about your steps or even look at the pedometer at all during the day; just ignore it. Each night write down that day's total number of steps (not miles or calories—just focus on steps) and then reset the pedometer to zero for the next day.

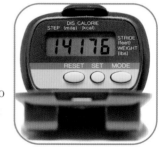

At the end of a week, add up the seven days and divide by seven, thus calculating your average daily steps—what we call a baseline activity level. Now multiply that number by 1.2 (a 20 percent increase) to calculate your daily target for the second week. So, let's say in the first week you found you averaged about 3,000 steps per day—not uncommon for someone who drives to work and sits at a desk all day, for example. Your goal in the second week would be to target 3,600 steps a day. That's a 20 percent increase, and a total of about five minutes of walking at a typical 120-step-per-minute (roughly 3 mph) pace. Each week that you successfully attain your average, boost your goal 20 percent again. If you fall short, then simply try to hit that week's target again.

How long should you keep going? Initially just focus on 20 percent weekly increases. But over time try to work up to averaging 10,000 steps per day. That's an activity level that roughly compares to getting thirty minutes of moderate daily activity, and it's been shown in a number of research studies to help people maintain a healthy weight and overall level of good health. The advantage of a pedometer is that you get credit for activity throughout your day rather than having to find 30 minutes or more all at once.

Substitute active for inactive time

Dr. Andrea Dunn, coauthor of *Active Living Every Day*, has done some intriguing studies of what it takes to help people start and maintain more active lifestyles. One of her findings is that some people find it easier to reduce the inactive time in their day, as opposed to focusing only on creating more active time. Specifically, Dr. Dunn feels replacing slothful parts of your day with more energetic options dramatically improves the likelihood of success.

Here are some easy ways to get in more active time (and log more steps on your pedometer) in a day:

1. Use a bathroom on another floor at work or school.
2. Get a post office box and walk to pick up the mail.
3. Choose to go to a more distant cafeteria or restaurant for lunch; if you make your own lunch, walk to a park or mall to eat.
4. Walk to a corner store for the newspaper, milk, or bread.
5. Carpool with a friend and walk to her house for the ride.
6. Occasionally skip e-mail and hand-deliver messages to people.
7. Walk the kids to school, a friend's house, or soccer practice rather than driving them (they'll end up healthier, too)!
8. Take a quick stroll rather than sit down for a midmorning snack.

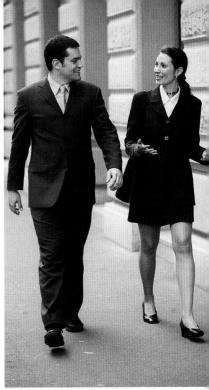

CALIBRATE YOUR PEDOMETER

Pedometers were originally designed as devices to estimate the distance you walk. If you'd like to estimate distance with your pedometer, calibrate it by wearing it while walking a known distance, like once around a quarter-mile track, at your normal walking speed. Then multiply your number of steps by 4 and you'll know your typical number of steps per mile. (For greater accuracy, you could simply walk a full mile—four times around the track.) Anytime you want to estimate the distance you've walked, just divide the total number of steps you've taken by your steps-per-mile calibration. Keep in mind that this is just an estimate, because the length of your stride increases as you speed up; on faster walks you'll be underestimating somewhat, and on slower walks you'll overestimate a bit.

Some pedometers allow you to enter your step length (based on a calibration walk); they'll calculate your walking distance automatically. Fancier models will even estimate the calories you burn if you enter your body weight as well. But don't count on these calorie estimates to be particularly accurate, given the wide variation of fitness levels and personal physiology of individuals.

Here's an example: Jan wears her pedometer for a walk around the 0.25-mile school track—it counts 473 steps. She multiplies by 4 to estimate that she takes about 1,892 steps a mile. (For easier math, she calls it 1,900 steps.) The next day she takes a walk and covers 6,685 steps. Jan divides 6,685 by 1,900 to get 3.52, or about 3.5 miles walked.

To calculate your step length, divide the known distance you've walked in feet by the number of steps you've taken. A 0.25-mile walk is 1,320 feet long (a mile is 5,280 feet). So Jan divides 1,320 feet by her 473 steps and learns that each step is 2.79 feet long. Now she can enter this into her pedometer.

Break it up

Which is better for you: walking 30 minutes all at once, or walking 10 minutes three times during the day? This is a trick question.

Breaking your 30 minutes of exercise into smaller chunks of time over the day provides the same health benefits. This is good news for lots of new walkers. Whether you walk 30 minutes all at once, or 10 minutes on the way to work in the morning, 10 minutes at lunch, and 10 minutes in the evening, over the long run you should see similar improvements in cholesterol levels and blood pressure, cardiovascular risk, and weight loss. Thus, if you're having trouble getting organized for a full 20- or 30-minute walk, break it up.

Walk Talk: Can I count little bits of activity—just a few minutes' worth, say—toward my daily walking total?

Exercise researchers will tell you that 8 to 10 minutes is the shortest exercise bout that has been studied; they're just not sure of the value of anything shorter. Some experts are suggesting, however, that even little doses of movement such as pacing while you're talking on the phone rather than sitting down, or fidgeting while you're standing in an airport line rather than sitting on your luggage, can add up over the course of the day. Their idea is that if you move enough to increase the total calories you expend in a day, it's probably good for you.

A number of recent articles on pedometers confirm the idea that activity spread throughout the day offers health benefits. For example, women in a six-month study, who increased their daily steps from 5,400 to 9,700, averaged an 11-point drop in systolic blood pressure and lost three pounds.

Spread the word

Dr. Dunn would call this enlisting support, and it's a proven strategy in helping people create a more active life. It's as simple as this: Tell anyone and everyone you know that you're walking, and ask for their help. Mention it at work, the dinner table, parties, everywhere. This will have two effects. First, the next time people see you, they'll ask how your walking is going. Second, and more important, you're likely to run across people who would like to join you occasionally. Walking with a partner has been shown to increase the chances that you'll stick with your walking.

Even if they can't walk with you, people are likely to be helpful as you make time for your walks if you're clear that this is a priority for you. Perhaps your spouse will pick up the kids, or coworkers will understand if you'd rather not do a lunch meeting because that's when you walk. Maybe the kids will even clean up after supper! (Well, you can dream, can't you?)

Map out opportunities

One exercise that Dr. Dunn leads with the folks she has counseled involves a detailed map of your local area and a string. (A local real estate map might work well.) Cut the string to the length of 1 mile on the map's scale and use it to draw a circle with a 1-mile radius—that's a 15- to 20-minute walk—centered on your home. Then mark on the map the places where your friends and your children's friends live, stores, parks where you can take your dog—anything that gives you a chance to get in some of your walking. Post the map on your refrigerator as a reminder of all the places you might travel to on foot now that you're building an active lifestyle.

Log it

It's a fact that people who keep a log show a greater chance of sticking with exercise than those who don't. That said, there is no single or right way to keep a log. Left to their own devices, everyone comes up with a slightly different, individualized approach to keeping an exercise diary. Some walkers have elaborate logbooks designed specifically for recording daily exercise, with specific locations for noting distance and time walked plus strength, flexibility, and other activities. Others use a simple monthly calendar that also houses other household appointments and schedules, and they just write their walking time in the lower corner of each date box. There are some universal ingredients in successful exercise logs, however.

TIPS FOR AN EXERCISE LOG

• **Keep it accessible.** Some walkers keep a logbook on their bedside table, others in their purse or brief-case, and still others post it in a prominent place, such as on the family calendar. Wherever you put your log, try to make it high profile so you see it often. Keep it there all the time so you always know where to find it.

• **Set up a system.** The more complicated your log, the harder it is to maintain. Have a simple system—always write the time you walked in one place, how you felt in another. One of my friends uses a red pen to note his walking mileage each day. It's the only thing he writes in red. This way, he can assess his weekly walking mileage with just a quick scan. Create a simple format of your own, and be consistent so it's easy to look back and find things.

• **Don't write too much.** Specifically, don't record any more than you're likely to be interested in reading later. Certainly, information such as how far you walked and how you felt is worthwhile—it helps you measure your progress. But over time, try to notice what's helpful and what's extraneous.

• **Keep a running tally of mileage.** The single thing walkers like most about an exercise log is seeing how many walking miles they've accumulated over time. It makes their success very concrete and palpable. It's easiest if you jot down an estimate of the miles you walk each day, then keep a running total, simply adding each day to your current total for the year. It's also worth noting and comparing weekly mileage totals, to catch any sudden increases or drops.

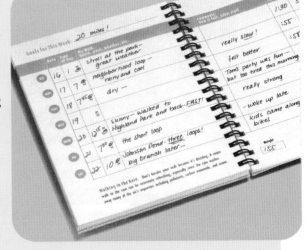

• **Look back at your log once in a while.** One goal of a log is to help you learn from your experience. So noting places or routes you've enjoyed, or food that doesn't sit well on a long walk, can be very educational. It can also help you figure out the cause of a particular problem. Could your shins be sore because of a sudden increase in weekly mileage, or more workouts than usual on hills? A log can help, but only if you look back at it now and then.

Lock it in

Setting your walking time just like any other appointment in your day is a great way to deal with that common complaint, "I don't have enough time for exercise." Many successful walkers say they write the time for their walks in their daily calendar or to-do list, even if it's just a 15-minute walk. They also say it's one of the most satisfying things to check off when they're done, because they invariably feel better after their walk than they did before.

Even more powerful than simply setting the time is to have the appointment with another walker. My friend Betsy, who has a very demanding schedule at the Denver public television station, gets up at 5:30 every day to walk. She has an appointment to walk at that time with two neighbors, and they signal that they're ready to go by turning on certain lights in their houses for the others to see. Betsy says she's convinced that this appointment makes her get out there. Walking with others turns what would be a 30-minute obligation into an enjoyable 60-minute start to the day.

Combine "locking it in" with enlisting support and you've got a walk that's almost certain to happen.

Join the team

A formal, or even informal, walking club or team is a great way to make your walking more fun and more likely to happen. Walking organizations range from structured to casual, from competitive to social, and most are delighted to have new members. Here are a few types of clubs you might find (check out "Clubs and Walking Organizations" in the resource list at the end of this book):

• **Fitness walking.** Many of these groups hold weekly get-togethers to walk, sometimes in new locations. They're often based at health clubs, community centers, YMCAs, malls, and local park and recreation departments, so contact these entities in your area.

• **Racewalking.** These groups invariably welcome newcomers and are happy to teach absolute novices. They often gather for weekly workouts at a track, and many organize occasional races as much for fun as for competition. Some also organize more serious teams for regional and national competition. (See "Racewalking" in the resource list.)

• **Outdoor and hiking.** There are myriad local groups associated with a specific trail or wilderness area, and they often take on a stewardship role on trails or public lands as well as organizing group hikes. (See "Hiking" in the resource list.)

• **Informal groups.** Some of the most effective "clubs" I've seen are informal groups of walkers who live near one another and get together for regular walks. If nothing else, rustle up some friends for your own neighborhood club, and set a specific time and day for a once-a-week walk.

Set a goal

Although this is at the "structured" end of my list of motivational ideas, it's really a powerful tool, and everyone should give it a try. Behavioral researchers say that goal setting helps people create concrete targets for their exercise and makes it much easier to focus and feel successful. I also think it can be just plain fun.

A goal can be anything from training for a specific occasion or event to simply trying to walk a certain number of days in row. (See chapter 16 for information on lots of walking events, including

Walk Talk: Quick answers to the most common excuses not to exercise.

Excuse: I haven't exercised since junior high gym class.

Answer: Remember that you're not alone—almost a third of Americans are largely sedentary. So call an old friend from junior high and ask him to take a walk with you—he may need a walk as much as you!

Excuse: Exercise is boring.

Answer: Consciously make it fun. Consider joining a club or team so you'll have group workouts or events to join. Or—much simpler—try putting a treadmill in front of the television and walking while you watch the news. Whatever gets you moving.

Excuse: This is going to hurt.

Answer: Go back to the "Four-Week Warm-Up Program" on page 3 and try it first. Remember, it starts with 10-minute strolls, and you can do them at whatever pace is most comfortable for you—even stopping to rest if you need to.

Excuse: I weigh too much.

Answer: All the more reason to start now! Remember that if you're heavy, even small increases in your activity level will start to burn serious calories and begin revving up your metabolism. Consider multiple shorter walks rather than a single long one.

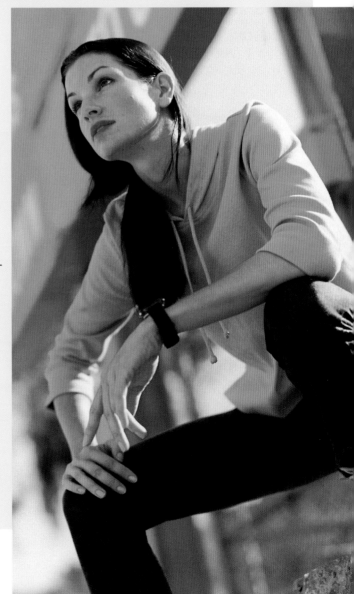

Excuse: I don't have the time.

Answer: It seems you never have the time until you make it. Try mapping out your daily travel and looking for opportunities for activity in the things you already do. Also, get a training log and use it like an appointment book, actually scheduling your walk as if it were a 15-minute meeting.

Excuse: I don't know where to start.

Answer: This program is your guide. Your problem may be starting alone—try talking to family and friends about embarking on this program, and see if you can recruit a regular partner. Then start a streak—a series of days with at least a 10-minute walk.

Excuse: It's raining out. It's too hot. It's too cold.

Answer: Humans have survived ice ages; you can walk in the rain. Just be sure to gear up so you're comfortable. If you're afraid of melting, seek out indoor options like malls or a treadmill. (See chapter 5 for gear and treadmill tips—it's the anti-excuse chapter.)

picking one suited to your personality and ability.) It's best if you have both a short-term and a long-term goal, but when you're just starting out, the short-term goal may be more important. Don't fixate right now on a goal like losing 20 pounds—that could still be months away. Instead go for immediate gratification, like knowing that if you just walk five days this week you'll start feeling better and sleeping better by the week's end. And promise yourself a reward if you meet your goal; this will make it much more likely that you'll do so.

It's easy to end up focusing on external motivators: a nagging spouse, say, or the way others perceive your weight or appearance. But in order to really make your walking program work, you'll have to make your goals internal—things that matter to *you*, not anyone else. So focus on why you're walking—how much better you feel, or activities that your growing fitness makes more enjoyable.

The gift that keeps giving

Whether you are super-structured and go out for a walk at the same time every day, or you're totally flexible, wear a pedometer, and sprinkle in additional steps throughout your day, know that the benefits of being more active start early and just keep coming.

The benefits of increased physical activity . . .

Within days:
- Reduced stress levels during and following activity.
- Lower blood pressure after a walk.
- Better sleep on more active days.
- Satisfaction in doing something good for yourself.

Within weeks:
- Generally improved mood.
- Less stiffness, fewer aches and pains.
- First measurable fitness improvements.
- Growing confidence; interest in better nutrition.

Within months:
- Modest but measurable, sustainable weight loss.
- Firming and toning of muscles.
- Improved fitness and metabolic measures.
- Greater "self-efficacy"—belief that you can and will succeed.
- Overall interest in a healthier lifestyle.

4

Building a Body for **Walking**

Is walking enough?

Building a regular daily walking habit is the first and most important step toward reaching long-term health. But you really should add two more elements if you want your program to be completely rounded: a modest routine of regular stretching and some strength training. I'll introduce a complete strength-training program in chapter 10, but for now here are three simple core exercises for posture and back health. As for the stretching, I truly mean a modest amount. Even though most exercise experts agree that you should stretch practically every day to help your muscles and joints maintain their healthy, natural range of movement, most also agree that just a few minutes is enough.

A simple stretching routine

During my last year as a competitive racewalker, I had started working full time. I was no longer the Spartan athlete living at the Olympic Training Center with few obligations and literally hours to devote to my training each day. As I started to feel the real-world time crunch, I began cutting things out of my training routines. One mistake I often made was allowing myself to skip my normal post-workout stretching routine. The result was a chronically sore hamstring that took years to finally restore to health. Interestingly enough, I eventually learned that it wasn't how much time I devoted to stretching that made a difference, but simply the fact of doing it practically every day.

Most coaches and therapists agree that regular, modest stretching—as little as a few minutes after every walk—can help you maintain the full range of movement in your joints and stave off the stiffness that often comes with years of repetitive exercise, or lack of exercise. Beginning on page 42 are three simple stretches that take just four minutes after every walk. All are done standing, so you can even do them in your work clothes after a commuting or lunchtime walk. In nice weather I often do them on the deck of the ferry that I take home from work in Boston, after my brisk walk to the dock.

Here are four tips for doing these or any stretches correctly:

1. **Stretch only warm muscles.** Stretching cold muscles can cause pain or injury, and won't be as effective as when muscles are well warmed up. So it's best to stretch after your walk, when your muscles are warmest and most compliant. If you prefer to stretch first, walk easily for at least 5 to 10 minutes to warm up, then stretch.

2. **Never bounce.** Gently hold the stretch position for about 10 to 20 seconds—instead of counting, try taking six or seven slow, deep breaths, and imagine exhaling muscle tension.

3. **Soften your knees.** Locking your knees can put a lot of strain behind the knee and on the lower back, so always keep the knees at least slightly bent.

4. **Don't wince.** Never push far enough that it causes a grimace; you should feel only a gentle stretch, and never any pain.

Four-minute after-walking stretch routine

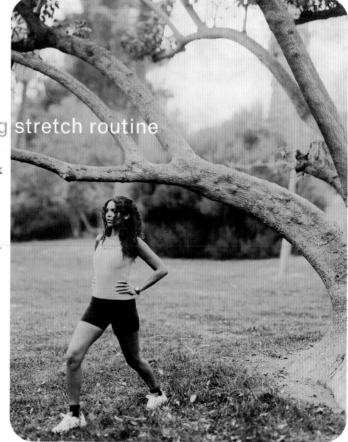

Do all of these stretches slowly, never to the point of discomfort; hold each stretch for six to eight slow, deep breaths. Begin each standing upright, and feel free to rest one hand on something for balance if necessary. If you have time, go through the cycle twice.

1. **Calf and hip.** Take a giant step forward with your right foot. Bend your right knee (but don't push it beyond your foot), keeping your left heel on the ground and your left leg straight behind you. Feel the stretch in both your left calf *and* hip. Hold. Then switch legs and repeat.

2. **Back and hamstring.** Stand with your feet together and your knees soft (not locked). Lean forward from the waist and let your arms and head hang loosely toward the ground. It's not necessary to touch your toes—just feel your body ease into the stretch with each deep breath. Slowly stand up and repeat.

3. **Shin and thigh.** Pull your left toes up behind you with your right hand, keeping your left knee pointed toward the ground. Your heel doesn't have to reach your buttocks—just pull to the point of feeling a gentle stretch in the hip, thigh, and shin. Hold, then switch legs and repeat.

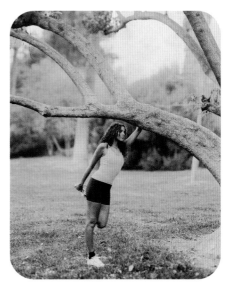

Walk Talk: Does my walking technique make any difference at all?

Yes, walking technique really does matter—and your first goal should be to get your posture in line. A tall body is more efficient and powerful, and less prone to discomfort. To get it right, focus your eyes on the horizon and feel like a string is pulling you up at the top of your head. Keep your shoulders back, not rolled forward, and gently contract your abdominal muscles to avoid what I delicately call shelf-butt—an excessive arch in your lower back and the protruding buttocks that go with it.

This efficient walking posture is especially important when you're carrying a baby pack or pushing a stroller. Both are likely to make you hunch your shoulders or lean forward from the hips, which can reduce your efficiency and add to lower-back strain. So remember to walk tall—try keeping only one hand on the stroller when you can, to reduce the chance of leaning on it too heavily.

Keep in mind that this should be your posture all the time, not just while walking. Constantly think about tall posture and taking the slouch out of your back, whether you're carrying groceries, typing on the computer, or driving the car. And make the quick core torso strengtheners beginning on page 44 a regular part of your routine just a few days a week—to really help this stick.

Building core strength

It is vitally important to keep your spine and torso strong. This is the basis of good posture not just while walking, but also in everything you do. Three simple exercises can challenge the front, back, and side muscles that stabilize your spine while offering the least risk of lower-back discomfort—a common complaint following traditional ballistic sit-ups.

I recommend adding the 10-minute routine below to your after-walk stretches (or doing them any other time they're convenient) two to four days a week. It will both firm and flatten your tummy as well as help with your posture. It also provides a quick and efficient overall strength-building program to complement your walking.

Three-move core strength routine

1. Curl-ups.

- Lie on your back with one knee bent, the other straight (both feet on the floor), and your hands flat below the small of your back.

- Tighten your stomach so you curl up, lifting your head, shoulders, and upper torso off the floor. Keep your gaze on a point above you on the ceiling so your neck stays relaxed.

- Hold the up position for a moment, then relax.

- After 5 repetitions, switch the straight and bent legs.

- Start with as few as 10 curl-ups at a time, but work up to 20 or 30 in a row, with all your movements slow and controlled.

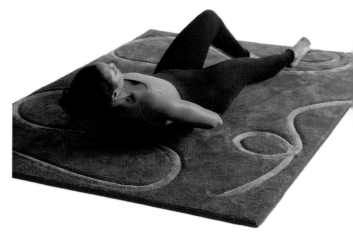

2. Isometric side support.

- Lie on your right side with your body straight and your left shoulder directly above your right, left hip above the right.

- Lift your body, supporting yourself only on your right elbow, forearm, and foot. Keep your left arm lying on your straight body.

- Hold for 5 to 10 seconds, breathing slowly and deeply, then rest and switch sides.

- Work up to several supports on each side.

- To make these easier, place your upper hand on your lower shoulder to distribute your weight more easily. Or bend your knees at a right angle and support yourself only from knees (not feet) to elbows.

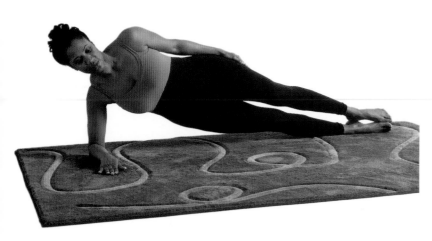

3. Alternate extensions.

- Start on your hands and knees, and lift your left leg out straight behind you.
- Hold for five seconds, relax, and switch legs.
- After 3 lifts on each side, when lifting your leg also hold the *opposite* arm out straight in front of you, for 3 more repetitions.
- Over time, build to doing up to 10 lifts on each side.

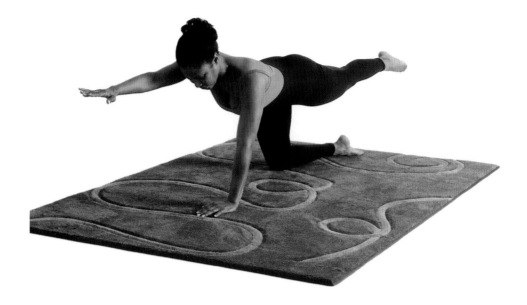

Walk Talk: How do I start toning my upper body, too?

It's a good idea to build your exercise program gradually. Over the first 16 weeks of the walking program, you'll regularly incorporate the stretches and core strengtheners described in this chapter, plus you'll continue boosting your walking time. Keep in mind that most of the moves already mentioned are for your full body, and they'll be helping build your overall strength and muscle tone, including your upper body. For example, the alternate-extension exercise involves the muscles of the arms, shoulders, and back, which you'll recognize very clearly after doing several repetitions.

But one very simple do-anywhere exercise you can add to begin focusing specifically on the upper body is the wall press:
- Stand an arm's length away from a wall and place your hands on the wall several inches below shoulder height, shoulder-width apart.
- Bend your elbows and, keeping your body straight from ankles to shoulders, lean in until your head almost touches the wall.
- Keeping your body stiff as a board from head to toe, straighten your arms and press back so that you're standing upright.

Begin with 5 to 10 repetitions, and build up to 15. As you get stronger, you can move your feet farther from the wall and place your hands a bit lower, so that your forward lean is greater. Eventually, you can move to doing presses off the back of a heavy couch or park bench.

	Date	Today's Activity Goal(s)	Total Minutes (or √)	Stretch? (√)	Comments, Other Activities? (vigorous chores, sports, other exercise, etc.)	Estimated Miles Walked
Sunday		20				
Monday		25				
Tuesday		15				
Wednesday		20				
Thursday		30				
Friday		off				
Saturday		40				

Miles this week: _____

Total miles for the year: _____

Recruit a walking partner—or a few

Some of the most successful long-term walkers I've met walk with others on a regular basis. (It's no surprise that research has proven people who exercise with others tend to be more successful, too.) To call them "informal clubs" doesn't do many of these groups justice. They don't have dues or formal club meetings, but their members walk together religiously and provide critical support, through the worst weather and even through personal difficulties.

Tip for the week. Invite a spouse, parent, child, sibling, friend, professional colleague, or even the last person to tell you a really good joke out to walk with you. If you enjoy yourselves, make a specific plan to walk together again—set a time and a place, and write it down in your log so you don't forget. Strive to make it a regular walking date.

Date	Today's Activity Goal(s)	Total Minutes (or √)	Stretch? (√)	Comments, Other Activities? (vigorous chores, sports, other exercise, etc.)	Estimated Miles Walked
Sunday	20, core				
Monday	25				
Tuesday	20				
Wednesday	20, core				
Thursday	30				
Friday	off				
Saturday	45				

Miles this week: _____

Total miles for the year: _____

Add the core strength routine twice a week

A three-exercise core strength routine consisting of an abdominal crunch, isometric side support, and alternate arm-and-leg extension is introduced in chapter 4. The good news is that the exercises are a lot simpler than their names. They're three simple moves you do on a carpet or exercise mat, and they'll help firm and flatten your abdominal and external oblique muscles (basically the middle and sides of your stomach), and strengthen your back, trunk, shoulders, and hips. (You'll find these core strength exercises on page 44.)

Tip for the week. Try to do the core strength routine at least twice a week. It's a critical step in maintaining healthy posture and preventing back pain. But introduce the exercises very gently—for the first three weeks, do much less than you think you're capable of, then increase gradually.

	Date	Today's Activity Goal(s)	Total Minutes (or √)	Stretch? (√)	Comments, Other Activities? (vigorous chores, sports, other exercise, etc.)	Estimated Miles Walked
Sunday		20, core				
Monday		30				
Tuesday		20				
Wednesday		20, core				
Thursday		35				
Friday		off				
Saturday		45				

Miles this week: _____

Total miles for the year: _____

Add a little—more or less—each week

If you're a detail person, you may have noticed that you're adding about 10 minutes of walking each week. It's a very gradual rate, which assures that you avoid injury and soreness, and it doesn't require massive lifestyle changes from one week to the next. But the time does pile up. In the first weeks you walked a total of barely an hour and a half; now you're almost up to three hours (the surgeon general's recommendation).

Tip for the week. This is just a reminder that to remain healthy and get the best workout, you have to use your best walking technique. Walk tall with your eyes looking forward, not at the ground, and focus on a quick, comfortable stride. You know you're doing it right if you have your eyes on the horizon.

Date	Today's Activity Goal(s)	Total Minutes (or √)	Stretch? (√)	Comments, Other Activities? (vigorous chores, sports, other exercise, etc.)	Estimated Miles Walked
Sunday	20, core				
Monday	30				
Tuesday	20				
Wednesday	20, core				
Thursday	35				
Friday	off				
Saturday	50				

Miles this week: ———————

Total miles for the year: ———————

Keep up the stretching habit

"Uh-oh," you're thinking, "I've got to stretch, I've got to do the core exercises, I've got daily walks. I can see where this is headed, and I can't do it all." Time for a quick perspective check.

First, when in doubt, walk. That's most important; it's your overall fitness builder and metabolism booster.

Second, commit to just four minutes of stretching after every stroll—it can help keep your joints supple and healthy for tomorrow's walk.

Third, the core strength routine is critical to your overall strength, posture, and (especially) bone and back health. It takes just 10 to 15 minutes two days a week, and is well worth the investment.

Tip for the week. **Remember your priorities. A daily walk is most important, and must happen even on your busiest days. Add a few minutes of stretching whenever possible; on your most relaxed days add the strength routine.**

	Date	Today's Activity Goal(s)	Total Minutes (or √)	Stretch? (√)	Comments, Other Activities? (vigorous chores, sports, other exercise, etc.)	Estimated Miles Walked
Sunday		20, core				
Monday		35				
Tuesday		20, core				
Wednesday		25				
Thursday		35, core				
Friday		off				
Saturday		50				

Miles this week: _____

Total miles for the year: _____

Increase the core strength routine to three days

Now that you're familiar with the core exercise routine, you can probably finish all three moves in just about 10 minutes. You're also probably feeling a little stronger—firmer through the stomach and more comfortable holding good, tall posture with your head up and shoulders back. As you master fitting this routine into your schedule, begin adding a third day of it to the week.

Tip for the week. **Try different times of day for the core strength routine. Here are three times that might work well:**
1. **First thing in the morning, before you even get cleaned up and dressed for the day.**
2. **Right after your walk, when you're already warmed up.**
3. **In the evening in front of the television.**

	Date	Today's Activity Goal(s)	Total Minutes (or √)	Stretch? (√)	Comments, Other Activities? (vigorous chores, sports, other exercise, etc.)	Estimated Miles Walked
Sunday		20, core				
Monday		35				
Tuesday		20, core				
Wednesday		30				
Thursday		35, core				
Friday		off				
Saturday		55				

Miles this week: _____

Total miles for the year: _____

Let your walks do some work for you

Your weekday walks are regularly surpassing 30 minutes now, and the longer weekend walks are approaching an hour. That's enough time for a comfortable 2- to 4-mile round-trip walk, which should make going places and doing errands on foot more reasonable. So try to replace at least one trip a week that you normally take in the car with a trip on foot instead. Already doing it? Then start working on an entirely car-free day!

Tip for the week. **Search out stores, services, and automatic teller machines that are within walking distance of where you live and work. Worried that they're more expensive than the stores you normally drive to? Look at it this way: Spending a few cents more on a gallon of milk at the corner store is nothing compared to the cost of a health club membership. And don't forget to factor in the money you're saving on gasoline.**

	Date	Today's Activity Goal(s)	Total Minutes (or √)	Stretch? (√)	Comments, Other Activities? (vigorous chores, sports, other exercise, etc.)	Estimated Miles Walked
Sunday		20, core				
Monday		40				
Tuesday		20, core				
Wednesday		30				
Thursday		40, core				
Friday		off				
Saturday		55				

Miles this week: _____

Total miles for the year: _____

If you do nothing more, maintain this routine for the rest of your life

Well, you've done it. If you do all the recommended walks and exercises this week, you'll be exceeding the surgeon general's advice to get at least 30 minutes of activity most days of the week. In fact, with the daily stretching and three days of the core strength routine, you're a veritable exercise dynamo! Remember this—even if you don't increase another step and don't speed up a bit, you'll be at a reduced risk of cardiovascular disease, diabetes, osteoporosis, obesity, and even some cancers if you just keep this up. This modest investment of just over three hours of activity a week is the best investment you could ever make.

Tip for the week. No matter how much farther you go in the program, set a routine like this week's in your mind as your minimum goal. Then even when you're busy or life is in turmoil, you'll know what your "default" activity level should be.

Date	Today's Activity Goal(s)	Total Minutes (or √)	Stretch? (√)	Comments, Other Activities? (vigorous chores, sports, other exercise, etc.)	Estimated Miles Walked
Sunday	20, core				
Monday	40				
Tuesday	20, core				
Wednesday	30				
Thursday	40, core				
Friday	off				
Saturday	1:00				

Miles this week: _____

Total miles for the year: _____

Has your habit improved? Check your progress

Look back over your log and count how many days you've walked in the past eight weeks. Check your score on the list in week 8 (see page 28), and compare to how you did in the first eight weeks. Also look for these key signs of success:

• You see an improvement in days walked. Walking more days shows you're mastering the art of building walking into your life.
• You're stretching regularly. A sign of dedication, but it also suggests a reduced risk of injuries and better preparation for moving on in the program.
• You do the core strength routine at least twice a week. That's enough for overall health, and sets you up for more strength and toning in future weeks.

Tip for the week. **If you're doing worse than the first eight weeks, it's time to take a look at what's changed in life. Job tension? Unsupportive family? Harder courses at school? Or is the novelty just wearing off? Tackle the problem directly—and if it's boredom, try ramping up to prepare for a hike in the next eight weeks of the program.**

5

Gearing Up to Get Walking

Minimizing the barriers you face to getting out and walking every day will help your daily walk become a habit. It's such an enjoyable way to spend time—it's not like I'm telling you to get your teeth cleaned every day!—that once you reduce the number of reasons you can't get out and walk, I think you'll find you really look forward to your daily outings. For beginners, two issues are common stumbling blocks: feeling you don't have the right gear ("I'm no jock—I don't even own workout clothes") and having young children at home ("I'm not getting a babysitter just so I can go for a walk"). I'd like to offer three solutions: clothing you're likely to already own, gear for bringing a child along, and tips for walking on a treadmill right at home (or at the gym).

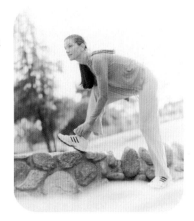

By the way, if pregnancy is the reason you're not walking, take a look at the "Walking Through Pregnancy" program in chapter 19. It takes you from nine months before the baby's birth to nine months after. (See page 223.)

You've got the gear to go

I think it's important to minimize any possible barriers to getting out the door and walking right away. Toward that end, I'd like to suggest that you probably have all the gear you need to start walking regularly right in your home. So for now, take a look in your closet and drawers and set up my super-economical exercise wardrobe.

The bottom layer: closest to your skin

If you've got fancy wicking undergarments like Cool-max or polypropylene, they're a great choice, because they transport moisture away from your skin if you work up a sweat. But for starters, any of your comfortable underwear—stuff you'd pick for working around the house on Saturday, not for going to a party—is fine. Avoid anything with itchy tags and tight spots.

For Women

Sports bras are the choice of many active women—some are comfortable, supportive, and discreet enough that it's all some women wear in very hot weather. They're largely a matter of personal choice and comfort, but keep in mind that more and more are available in moisture-wicking fabrics like Cool-max and polypropylene, which makes them even better suited to vigorous activity.

The middle layer: shirts and pants

Your focus should be on loose-fitting and comfortable garments. Your best-looking blue jeans are a bad call—they're probably way too tight. A pair of familiar khakis you're about ready to retire to gardening or a loose pair of shorts is more like it. Apply a similar comfort criterion for shirts. Or if you have a nylon or mixed-fabric sweat suit that you favor, that's fine. Cotton sweatpants and shirts are really suitable only for dry, cool days; keep in mind that if they get wet they become heavy and uncomfortable, and provide no insulation. Also, don't be afraid of some synthetics; synthetic materials will make clothes less clingy and damp if you break a sweat. Remember that this isn't a fashion show. Your goal is comfort.

The outer layer

The need for outer layers means it's either cold, wet, or both. For cold, nylon fleece materials (often called polar fleece) are the best insulators going. They're light, comfortable, and warm even when they're wet. You could soak a fleece jacket in water, squeeze it, shake it out, and wear it—and feel insulated. It may be a bit damp, but it's vastly better than a soaked cotton sweatshirt, which is essentially useless. If you don't have any fleece, then the original, natural alternative—wool—is a great choice.

I have a favorite wool sweater from Scotland (a gift from my wife) that I love on damp, cold walks along the ocean. It's a reminder of where the whole insulating-when-wet concept came from, and it has a dense, comforting feel and smell. Wear wool and you understand how sheep survive Scottish winters.

When wind and rain are threats, high-tech fabrics like Gore-Tex are great. They're designed to shed rain but allow sweat in the form of water vapor to escape the fabric. Don't panic if you don't own such fancy outerwear. For a 30-minute walk, a decent nylon windbreaker over your insulating layer will usually suffice in breaking the wind and withstanding a drizzle. In heavier rain I still like a good old rubberized slicker. A rain jacket and matching pants are inexpensive (as little as $35 for a set), and they keep you from using rain as an excuse not to take a walk. No, the fabric's not breathable, and on a longer or more vigorous walk dampness from within—your own sweat—can be a problem. But for a half hour at a moderate effort, it's perfect. Mine has a hood with a neat little brim to keep the rain drips off.

How about a hat?

I offer an unequivocal yes. I believe hats have three critical roles: protection from the sun in summer, insulation from the cold in winter, and defining your character as a walker year-round.

In summer the wider the brim, the better the sun protection you'll receive. In cold weather make sure your hat is thick and warm and covers your ears, since they're especially susceptible once the cold winds blow. As far as defining your character—that's just to encourage you to have a little fun in choosing your headwear.

Gloves

If it's just cool out, try walking with those inexpensive cotton gardening gloves. They're cheap, light, easy to stick in your pockets, and you're not distraught if you drop one by accident. If it's colder, I prefer light wool gloves, and densely knit wool mittens if it's really cold. Just keep in mind that though your core may stay warm when you're exercising, your hands can still chill quickly and make you uncomfortable. And you can always put gloves in your pockets if your hands warm up; you can't put them on if you haven't brought them along.

Socks

After shoes, I think that decent socks are next most important investment you can make. I prefer synthetic blends; cotton socks seem comfortable when warm and dry, but as soon as you sweat heavily in them they bunch up, lose cushioning, and can even cause blisters. Look for pairs with slightly thicker padding in the heel and ball of the foot (see "Socks" in the resource list at the end of this book).

Walking with children

One of the great appeals of walking is that it's an ideal activity for the entire family—not that all the members of the family will necessarily be walking under their own power. I've learned that having young children is absolutely no excuse not to maintain a daily walking habit. Quite the opposite, in fact. With the carriers and strollers now available, even those who aren't yet talkers can be avid walkers.

I've been doing some informal, unscientific research on parents and exercise habits when I take my son to his afternoon preschool. I'm divining two profiles. One is the stay-at-home parent who sees preschool as a long-awaited release—a few free hours to finally get personal things done, including exercise. Some parents even show up in exercise gear, ready to head to the gym or out for a walk. Many admit they've found it very hard to get regular exercise with small children in their lives.

Other parents involve exercise in their daily routine, and then bring their kids along for the fun. One example is a woman who regularly shows up on foot with her preschooler and a younger sibling in a nice all-terrain double stroller. She was active before she had children, and has made an effort to stay active. I'd like to think my wife Lisa and I fall into this second category. We found that especially right after the births of both of our children, daily walks were one of the ways we could be sure everyone got a good dose of fresh air and some physical activity. Even through the winter (my son was born in October, my daughter in February), we all slept better on days when we'd gotten a chunk of outside time. And as the woman with the double stroller proves, the gear exists to make it entirely feasible.

Safety tips for walking with children

Because you're walking with a child, you have to pay special attention to safety. Here are some safety tips you should be sure to follow:

- Wear lots of retro-reflective material, not just bright colors. At dawn, dusk, and night make sure you and the child are covered with a decent amount of reflective material, like 3M Scotch-lite, that will be visible in car headlights.

- Use all of the straps or harnesses provided to secure your child in a carrier or stroller. They may seem extraneous—until you stumble for the first time. Then you'll see how important they are in keeping little Horatio from tumbling out.

- Follow the manufacturer's instructions. Set parking brakes on strollers when standing still, and never leave a child unattended. Also, always wear the wrist leash so the stroller can't be lost on a downhill; trust me, I know this from experience. (I caught the stroller and everything was fine, except for my nerves.)

- Never use a carrier or stroller while wearing in-line skates. No matter how accomplished you are, it's not worth risking a serious fall.

- Be very cautious about holding dogs on leashes while you're carrying or pushing a child. A friend was walking two large dogs while carrying a child in a front pack. The dogs became excited by a squirrel, and within an instant they had wrapped up his legs and pulled him over. Despite his best efforts, his child's head hit the ground and she suffered a fracture. Thankfully, both are absolutely fine now, but it's a reminder that dogs can be powerful and very swift when agitated.

Front carriers: when they're small

Front carriers are a wonderful way to begin walking with a newborn. They keep the baby close to your chest, where you feel you can offer complete protection. There are front carriers for even the smallest child. Most allow babies to ride facing in toward you when they're very small, and facing away so they can see where you're walking as they get older. (See "Child Carriers" in the resource list at the end of this book.)

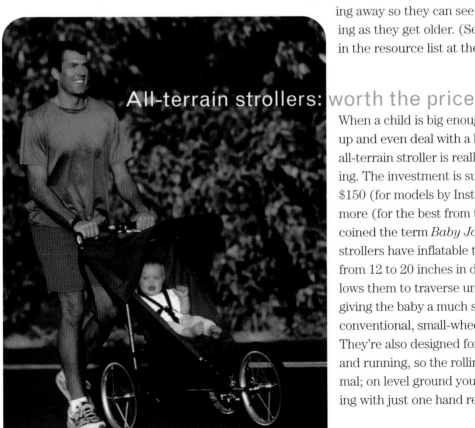

All-terrain strollers: worth the price

When a child is big enough to hold her head up and even deal with a bit of jostling, an all-terrain stroller is really worth considering. The investment is substantial, from $150 (for models by Instep) to $300 or more (for the best from the company that coined the term *Baby Jogger*). These strollers have inflatable tires that range from 12 to 20 inches in diameter, which allows them to traverse uneven terrain while giving the baby a much smoother ride than conventional, small-wheeled strollers. They're also designed for exercise walking and running, so the rolling friction is minimal; on level ground you can keep one moving with just one hand resting on the handlebar. Some models fold easily to fit into the trunk of a car, and add-ons like sun- and rain-screens and mosquito netting are available from various manufacturers. (See "Strollers" in the resource list.)

Backpacks:
big enough to take it all in

Once a child is strong enough to hold his head up, a backpack is the most versatile carrier going. You can wear it on the roughest terrain. Just keep in mind that you have a live load—someone who might squirm around to see some wildlife, or try to reach for his crackers or, I've found, even your hat. Also, remember that as the child gets taller, his head is as high as or even slightly higher than yours, so be very careful when passing under low-hanging branches. My wife was the self-designated, and very vocal, "low-bridge alarm" when I was carrying one of our children. Many of the models offer attachments ranging from rain and sun hoods to bottle carriers and extra carrying capacity under the child. (See "Child Carriers" in the resource list.)

Gear for indoors: the treadmill option

I'm a true believer that walking outdoors is perfectly reasonable in just about any season, anywhere in the United States. I feel somewhat justified in saying this, because I grew up in western New York State, between Rochester and Buffalo, a region known for harsh, gray winters and lots of snow. (Yes, that's the Buffalo you used to see on the news all the time setting snowfall records in the era before global warming.) I lived there long before they invented Gore-Tex, and I walked to school every day from fifth grade on. No, it wasn't uphill in both directions, and it was only 1.5 miles, but our superintendent prided himself on rarely canceling school. So I have little sympathy for healthy, able-bodied people telling me that they can't walk outside because of the weather.

There are some valid reasons, however, for occasionally not wanting to walk outdoors. They include safety concerns for a woman walking alone, dangerous traffic and the lack of sidewalks or pathways, the need to get in your walk while children are napping, difficult footing in winter for the elderly or unsteady, and even—yes, I'll admit it—severely cold weather. If you do find yourself unable to walk outdoors, you have two options: Find an indoor facility with enough space for walking, like a mall or a YMCA with an indoor track, or get on a treadmill.

Trying a treadmill

If you've never walked on a treadmill, I strongly recommend trying one before buying one. Some people enjoy a treadmill's consistency and safety for their walk practically every day. Others walk on a treadmill occasionally, say for bad weather, but they prefer walking outside. And still others, like me, would just as soon find a cross-training activity that involves boiling oil and sharp sticks before we'd walk on a treadmill. But that's a personal preference. The fact is, you can get a great workout on a treadmill in a perfectly safe, controlled environment.

You can test one at a gym or a YMCA. Many health clubs allow you one or two visits free if you're considering a membership; you'll have to sit through the full sales pitch, but it's a good way to see whether this setting might be a workout option for you and to give a treadmill a whirl. Or ask a friend if you can try hers for a couple of walks.

Walk Talk: How do I actually step onto a treadmill for the first time?

If you're an experienced treadmill walker, you may think this is a silly question. But that's just because you're forgetting the unsteadiness and hesitation you probably felt the first time you got onto a moving belt. After all, the ground is moving, you're actually standing still, and if you get it wrong you feel like the thing might just toss you right off the back. It's George Jetson and Astro all over again.

Fear not—treadmills are actually quite safe, and they're very easy to master. Here are a few tips for stepping onto a treadmill the first few times:

- Start by straddling the machine with one foot on each side of the belt and hands firmly on the handrails.
- Start the machine at a comfortable walking pace; not too slow, or it will feel unnatural to get on board. Try 2.5 miles per hour.
- Still holding the handrails, put just one foot on the moving belt several times, taking one-footed steps. You'll feel like you're pawing the belt. Then try it with the other foot.
- When you have a sense of the belt's speed, step on with both feet and begin walking, still holding the handrails. This is important—look forward, not down at your feet. You'll want to look down, but don't—it can make you unsteady.
- As you get used to looking forward, let go with one hand and let it swing normally. Then put it back and let the other hand swing free. Then keep only one hand very lightly on the handle, and finally let go entirely.
- Make sure you stand tall, look forward, and use your best walking technique. Don't worry about looking down to keep your feet on the belt. Use the handrails only to keep yourself centered and walking near the front of the machine.
- When it's time to stop, put one hand on the handrail and slow the 'mill to a saunter, then grab with both hands and straddle the machine before stopping it entirely. And be careful when stepping off the treadmill—you may feel unsteady for your first few steps on solid ground.

Treadmill workout ideas: whatever it takes

One shortcoming of walking on a treadmill is that the scenery never changes. Even worse, I see many people staring blankly at a television in a health club or reading a magazine as they walk. Here's the problem: Sauntering along at such a comfortable TV-watching or reading pace isn't likely to be much of a cardiovascular challenge. Which means you're not building much fitness.

It doesn't have to be that way, however. "A treadmill can be a perfectly good workout, as long as you take advantage of the machine's attributes. Utilize the speed and elevation adjustments to both make it more interesting and get a better workout," suggests Dave McGovern, a walking coach who travels the country giving clinics and coaching walkers from beginning fitness enthusiasts to accomplished athletes. (See "Instructors" in the resource list.) Here are a few simple treadmill workout ideas—more are offered in chapters 9 and 13.

Great treadmill workouts in 30 minutes or less

- **Speed up and down.**

The goal: Gently work up to your best cruising speed.

The workout: Begin walking at a comfortable pace, say 3 miles per hour, for eight minutes.

Then increase the speed by 0.2 miles per hour for two minutes; every two minutes add another 0.2 miles per hour. Stop increasing when you can hold the speed for only two minutes (or when you reach 4 miles per hour). Walk 2 minutes at this speed, then move back down, reducing by 0.2 miles per hour every two minutes, finishing up the 30 minutes at 3 miles per hour. If you successfully make it up to 4 miles per hour, then next time you do the workout start at 3.2 miles per hour and go up to 4.2 miles per hour; then try 3.4 miles per hour and so on.

- **The stair master.**

The goal: Developing thigh and buttock strength and tone.

The workout: If your treadmill's in the basement, this one's for you. After a 10-minute warm-up, alternate three minutes of brisk treadmill walking (3.5 to 4.5 miles per hour) with one minute of walking up and down a flight of stairs; repeat at least four times. Cool down at a comfortable pace.

- **The short circuit.**

The goal: A mix of aerobic and strength training that's guaranteed to boost your heart rate and strength.

The workout: After an 8-minute warm-up, walk at a brisk pace (3.8 to 4.5 miles per hour) for two minutes, then step off and do 30 seconds of a strength exercise, then get back on the treadmill for two minutes. Cycle through the three exercises of the core strength routine, plus the wall press (see chapter 4); do the routine twice. Don't dally getting on and off the machine to ensure that your heart remains challenged. Finish with five minutes of easy walking to cool down.

Selecting a treadmill

If you've tried some workouts on a treadmill and found them enjoyable, then it may be worth investing in your own machine. A weight-loss study reported in the *Journal of the American Medical Association* revealed that subjects who had a treadmill for use in their homes lost an average of four to eight more pounds than the subjects who didn't have treadmills. This may not seem like a huge difference, but given that the weight loss averaged only between 15 and 20 pounds over 6 months of the study, it's worth noting. Not surprisingly, the researchers felt one advantage of having a treadmill at home was that it was convenient to take several short walks rather than one long one each day.

A high-quality treadmill could easily cost $2,000 or more, though there are good machines available for less. The key is to match how you'll use the treadmill with its features. Don't buy what you don't need. Here are some things to consider when buying a treadmill:

- **How often will you use it?** If you'll fire up the machine practically every day, invest in heavy-duty hardware and go for all the features: automatic programs, calorie counters, maybe even a system that adjusts the treadmill speed to your heart-rate monitor's output to keep you in your target range. But if you know it's just going to be a backup for bad weather or hectic days, stick with a less elaborate machine.

- **What size is it?** Size matters. A lightweight and smaller walker may be able to comfortably use a less expensive, smaller machine, but in general look for at least an 18-inch-wide, 48-inch-long belt. Any less and you may be tempted to chop your stride unnaturally. Also, be sure to measure the ceiling height in the room you'll be using to make sure there will be adequate headroom even when the incline is maxed out.

- **Is speed in your future?** If you know you'll be ramping your walking up to serious speeds, or if you could imagine adding some running to your mix, invest in a heavier-duty model. Even if you never expect to walk faster than 5 or even 6 miles per hour, a machine rated to 8 or 10 miles per hour means you won't be testing its limits in your typical workout, and you'll have room to speed up as your fitness improves.

- **What's its incline?** An adjustable incline allows for greater variety and higher intensity in your workouts. Look for a 10 percent or greater incline if you intend to get in serious workouts on your machine. If it's just an emergency stop-gap, however, you can forgo this option.

Whatever you do, be sure to try before you buy. (You don't want to deal with any store that won't let you take a machine through its paces before buying.) Crank up the machine to its full speed and incline and make sure you have enough room and feel comfortable onboard. Also, find out if home delivery and assembly is an option—then you'll know your machine is up and running before the delivery person has even walked out the door.

BUYING POWER

Here are some more tips for a treadmill purchase:
- Look at the motor. Look for a motor that is continuous duty, and rated to at least 1.5 horsepower.
- Look at the deck. The belt should be long and wide enough for comfortable walking at highest speeds. Rollers should be at least 2 inches in diameter and solid; the larger the rollers, the smoother the ride.
- Listen for noise: Better-engineered treadmills make less noise but cost more. Lower-end models can drown out a television. Listen while you shop.
- Examine the warranty. Look for a lifetime warranty on the frame and two-year coverage on moving parts, motor, and electronics. A one-year labor warranty is also valuable. Avoid 90-day warranties if possible, and don't buy extended options; the basics should cover you.

Walk Talk: Can I consider buying a cheaper nonmotorized treadmill?

There are huge variations in the manufacturing and materials of exercise equipment. But because it's hardware-intensive, you largely get what you pay for. As a treadmill gets cheaper, you're likely to see less metal and more plastic, fewer welds and more screws, all of which stacks up to less durability. But for me, the real concern with nonmotorized treadmills is less workmanship than the nature of the workout. Nonmotorized machines require you to hold on to some sort of handle to keep your body in place while your feet move the belt. The result is that you may tend to be hunched over at the shoulders or leaning forward at the waist, which is far from your natural gait.

There are some interesting machines with levers that you pump in opposition to your legs while walking. The pumping action of your arms helps move the belt, so that the walking gait is somewhat more natural. But as far as I'm concerned, that's the standard to hold the machine to. Give it a full workout—30 minutes at least—and see if you can walk with a natural, upright posture for the full time and feel no tightness in your neck, shoulders, back, or buttocks. If so, then it's probably safe.

I suspect you'll find few nonmotorized models that meet this standard. If you do find one, then focus on its workmanship and materials, using the criteria I give for treadmill purchases in general. The bottom line is that if you're making the investment, it's worth investing in the best possible machine to meet your needs—it will pay off in the long walk.

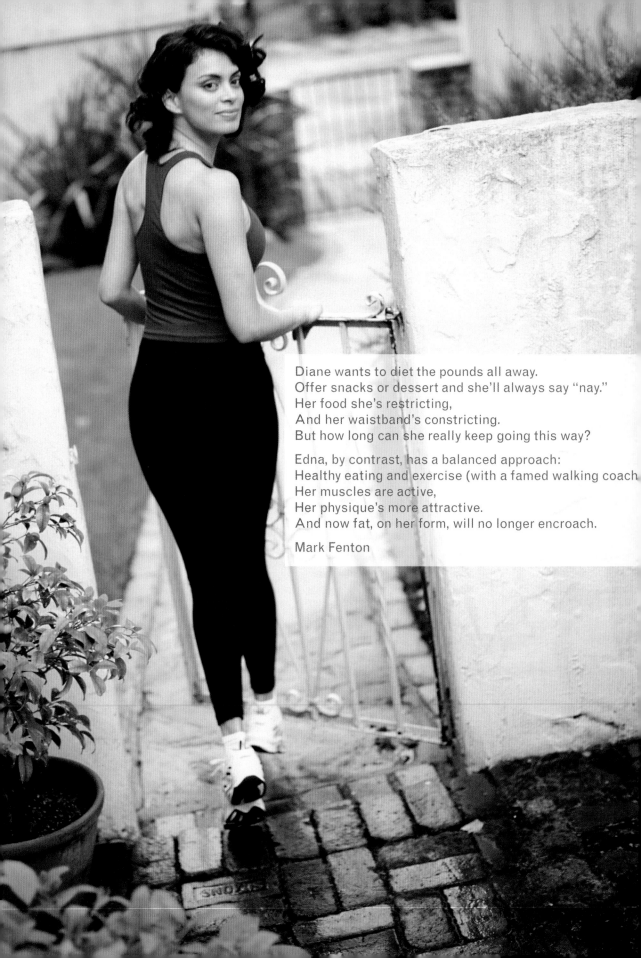

Diane wants to diet the pounds all away.
Offer snacks or dessert and she'll always say "nay."
Her food she's restricting,
And her waistband's constricting.
But how long can she really keep going this way?

Edna, by contrast, has a balanced approach:
Healthy eating and exercise (with a famed walking coach)
Her muscles are active,
Her physique's more attractive.
And now fat, on her form, will no longer encroach.

Mark Fenton

Part II

Walking for Weight Loss: Cranking Up the Metabolism and the Miles

[In New York City] you can't walk ten blocks in any direction without encountering shopfront extravaganzas of roasted meats, hand-made pastries, iced fishes, marzipans, pizzas, calzones, knishes, cannoli, kirschtortes, and a thousand other edible wonders. It's another irony that mainstream suburban America is full of diet-crazed fat people traveling about in cars, while New Yorkers walk off so many calories on a daily basis that they can eat great things with a clear conscience.

JAMES HOWARD KUNSTLER
HOME FROM NOWHERE, 1996

6

Weight Loss: The Great American Obsession

Do you know why you're walking? Is reduced stress and improved health enough for you, or do you really want to peel off some pounds? It's worth taking a moment to think about what your goals are and to be sure you're doing enough to meet them.

To help nail down your goals, take this quick quiz, "Setting Your Sights on Something." It's just three questions, but it will help you think about your exercise personality and why you're really walking.

QUIZ III
Setting Your Sights on Something

Which of these is most important for you?
   a) Long-term health and well-being and simply feeling better about myself.
   b) Improved health and well-being, but I also want to lose at least 10 pounds.
   c) I may want to lose a few pounds, and I certainly want to be healthy, but I really want to be more fit and strong and have a more athletic physique.

Which of the following vacations would you be most likely to take?
   a) A trip with lots of leisure time and relaxation, plus opportunities for walking tours of great museums or historic and natural sites to take as I please.
   b) A walking tour from inn to inn or town to town, with moderate daily walks and plenty of rest and relaxation in the evenings, and the option for some bike riding, too.
   c) A trekking vacation in the Canadian Rockies, or a visit to climb the volcanoes and shore trails of Hawaii, with some mountain biking or kayaking planned in the mix.

Which of these workouts would leave you feeling the best?
   a) A nice 30-minute walk outdoors, enjoying nature and the simple joy of moving.
   b) A brisk 40-minute stroll that leaves my muscles warm and me breathing noticeably, then a few minutes of relaxing stretching.
   c) A fast 35-minute walk that leaves me sweaty and breathing hard, followed by some weight lifting and stretching.

Score 1 point for an (a), 2 points for a (b), and 3 for a (c).

If you scored:

• **3 or 4 points.** You'll flourish in a program aimed at maintaining a *healthy mind and body*. The key for you is to balance your walking with just enough stretching and other activity to maintain muscle and bone health and to avoid injuries. The basic walking program introduced in part 1 of this book—weeks 1 through 16—may be sufficient for you, because you probably don't want exercise to become onerous or too demanding in your life. But you should also add some of the strength and cross-training lessons of part 2 and motivational lessons from part 3 to your routine. One approach: Try some of these lifestyle-based ideas to build incidental cross-training into your week beyond your daily walking.

Tactical tips:
• Plant a garden (big enough that it requires some digging and weeding).
• Purchase a nonmotorized push lawn mower and use it.
• Attend a weekly dance, or sign up for a once-a-week dance or aerobics class.
• Sign up to coach a children's soccer or basketball team—and hustle with the kids.
• Come up with any equally active chore or avocation and make it a habit.

• **5 to 7 points.** You seem well suited to a *fitness and weight-control program*. You'll benefit from boosting the length and speed of your walks occasionally to burn more calories and build more fitness; stick with the walking program in the book at least through week 32. Make regular stretching a habit, too, and add at least the simple at-home strength routine introduced in chapter 10. A mix of cross-training activities will also add to your success.

Tactical tips:
• Purchase a yoga, stretching, or tai chi video with 15- to 30-minute routines and use it once or twice a week.
• Buy a set of dumbbells (ranging from 3 to 10 pounds) for use at home so you'll have no excuse to skip the strength routine in this section of the book.
• Make two firm workout dates a week, ideally with a friend but at least with yourself. It's best to schedule your longest and fastest walks of the week, because they're the ones you want to be certain not to miss.

• **8 or 9 points.** You're ready to start striving for your *optimal performance*. You probably want a comprehensive program for building fitness, strength, coordination, and flexibility—including the walking and strength-training programs introduced in part 3 of this book. Keep in mind that high fitness demands a commitment equal to the task; you should certainly continue with the walking, strength, and cross-training program through week 48. But know that doing so will provide the best health profile and allow for such inherent variety in the walking and cross-training activities that it can be the most fun!

Tactical tips:
• Your key to success will be learning to do things correctly. From trying yoga to building a weight circuit routine, be sure to get instruction on anything new you do—it will reduce the chance of injury and increase the effectiveness of your workouts.
• Focus on proper fast-walking technique to really reach your highest speeds and greatest aerobic challenge.

- Begin all of your new activities gradually and patiently, giving yourself time to build strength and skill.
- Consider joining a health or racquet club or sports team to help lock in some of your cross-training activities.

Diane and Edna: a weight-loss story

I know two women, Diane and Edna. Neither of them currently exercises. They both want to lose weight, so they decide to be smart and go to a nutritionist for a dietary analysis. They estimate that they each eat about 2,000 calories a day. Their doctor (they also go to the same doctor) then tells them that they could safely drop their caloric intake to about 1,500 calories a day. This gets Diane and Edna very excited, because—as the doctor explains—if they reduce their net intake by 500 calories a day and maintain their current activity levels, they could lose a pound a week. That's because one pound of body fat equals about 3,500 calories of energy; dropping 500 calories seven days a week equals 3,500 calories a week. "Yippee," say Diane and Edna, "10 pounds off in 10 weeks!"

Diane decides to diet very carefully. She cuts out lots of fats, stops eating butter and all oils, won't even look at desserts, and successfully restricts herself to eating just 1,500 calories a day.

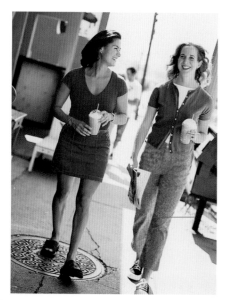

Edna, on the other, decides to start exercising along with eating a healthy diet. In fact, she averages a brisk 45-minute walk every day. Some days she goes a bit longer; others, shorter. To improve her diet, Edna starts eating more fruits and vegetables. She makes slight changes, such as substituting jelly on her bagel for cream cheese, but not nearly as significant as Diane. In fact, she manages to cut only 250 calories a day out of her diet. But get a load of this: Because her 45-minute walk burns about 250 calories a day, overall she and Diane are in about the same place. On *net* they both cut out about 500 calories a day. It's just that Diet Diane gets there by lopping 500 calories out of her diet, while Exercise Edna cuts 250 calories from what she eats and burns off another 250, for her net drop of 500.

Now let me ask you two simple questions: Who is likely to maintain this weight loss over time? More important, who is having more fun doing it?

In the beginning Diane and Edna will probably fare about the same. They'll both begin to lose about a pound a week, if all other things in their life (like normal daily activity) remain the same. But here's the catch: As they begin to lose weight, Diet Diane's body will begin to require fewer calories to stay alive. For example, if she drops from 150 to 140 pounds over 10 weeks, she might need to cut another 100 calories a day just to maintain her new lower weight. Even worse, research suggests that she won't just be losing fat as her weight drops—she is also likely to lose some muscle. *Effectively, Diane's metabolism is slowing down as she loses weight*, and she'll have to continue restricting her diet just to avoid future weight gain.

Exercise Edna, on the other hand, is using her muscles with her daily walks. So even though she'll lose 10 pounds, too, more of her lost weight will be fat, and she'll keep or even build some muscle. *Effectively, Edna's metabolism has been maintained or even increased with exercise.* Because she has more muscle mass to supply with energy than Diane does, she may be able to eat a little more on a daily basis and still maintain that lower weight.

As for the question of fun, is there even any doubt? Diane is restricting her diet more, may feel her energy is waning, and gets ticked off at how much she has to sacrifice to make progress. Sound familiar? Edna, on the other hand, is enjoying invigorating daily walks and feels healthier and more energetic than ever. With her newfound fitness, she'll also find her desire for more fattening and less nutritious foods diminishing—her active body will run better on healthier choices like whole grains, fruits, and vegetables.

Diet *and* exercise are the key

Diane and Edna are not figments of my imagination; they're composites. They represent the thousands of people I've talked to or who wrote to *WALKING* Magazine about their attempts at weight loss over the years. In every case two things are clear about people who have been successful:

1. They're not eating a fad diet—no low-carb/high-fat fiasco. Just more fruits and vegetables, whole grains, and lots of water. You could lock me in a room for a week with Dr. Atkins and I'll still say the same thing.
2. They walk every day, religiously. In fact, their walking is the foundation of their weight-loss success, even though their improved diet may be the greater lifestyle change.

Their stories are also consistent with weight-loss research that's been undertaken in recent decades. The key finding is this: For successful long-term weight loss, a program including a moderate, balanced diet and regular daily physical activity has the greatest chance of success. Can people lose lots of weight on highly restrictive diets alone? Yes. Have people successfully exercised away pounds without changing their diet at all? Certainly some have. But if you won't be satisfied losing 20 pounds now—in time, say, for your daughter's wedding—and then gaining it (and 5 pounds more!) back in eight months, you should be looking at a combination of balanced diet and regular exercise. This combination has repeatedly been shown to have the greatest chance to result in permanent weight loss.

Why weight matters

Imagine an ideal world in which people aren't obsessed with body size and shape. Instead, our greatest concern about our bodies would simply be wringing the most life out of them. We'd want the longest, healthiest, most energetic, active, adventurous lives our bodies could offer. We'd all find ways to express ourselves physically that suited our own physiques and psyches best. Some would dance, others would play sports; some would go to gyms, others would spend their days outside in physical labor; everyone, though, would experience the joy of regular physical activity. Of course everyone would walk, and no one would think about bathroom scale.

Dream on, Mark. We are a society obsessed by the bathroom scale—not entirely without reason. The medical evidence is clear that obesity is strongly related to chronic diseases, like diabetes and cardiovascular disease, and an early death. Just as debilitating may be the reduced quality of life that can accompany obesity—from physical limitations and sleep disorders to social stigmas and self-consciousness. Far from my dream of a culture that celebrates active, healthy living, instead we seem to celebrate the ideal of skinny, perfect bodies. This just adds to the difficulty of being heavy in our society.

What would I really like to see? I want society to stop wishing everyone were sickly-thin supermodels and start realizing it's time we took steps (many steps, most days of the week) toward reaching happier and healthier weights. The good news is that experts all agree on the solution: regular daily physical activity and a moderate, balanced diet. No insane workout regimen, no deprivation diets. Or as one phrase that reappears at every academic conference I attend goes: *Move a little more, eat a little less.*

The bathroom-sink theory (and the first law of thermodynamics)

One way to understand how diet and exercise work is to think of your body as a sink. No, not its shape; just think of it as a vessel into and out of which energy flows.

First, imagine the water flowing out of the spout and then on down the drain as being actual energy—energy measured in terms of calories. It's possible for the water to run straight through, just as it's possible for calories to enter your body (whenever you eat food) and flow right out (as you spend them going about your daily tasks).

Unfortunately, a backup can occur when more calories enter the sink than are able to travel on out the drain. Whenever you eat or drink, you're filling the sink. What types of foods you eat affect how quickly the sink fills. For instance, foods high in fat have more calories than basic carbohydrates—a gram of fat has about nine calories (lots of water to fill the sink), while a gram of carbohydrate has only about half that many (much less water in the sink). If you keep running water into the sink faster than it can drain, the sink will begin to fill, essentially storing the water until the sink has a chance to drain.

Storing extra energy

Just as the sink stores extra water, your body stores extra calories it's not using. Carbohydrates are turned into sugars and stored in "easy-access" places such as muscle cells, the bloodstream, and your liver. This sugar is easy to burn and ready to go whenever you need energy. It's just sitting there waiting for you to open the drain by being active so—swooooosh!—it can go flowing out.

However, once all the easy-access storage places are filled, your body starts storing extra energy as fat. Fat is a convenient high-density way for your body to store extra calories, and you tend to put it in all your favorite places: hips and thighs, belly, the back of your upper arms. Nice image, huh? A sink full of fat!

Of course, whenever you're physically active your body needs energy, so the drain opens wider to use some of the stored fuel. This is the act of burning calories. As long as you're alive, the drain is always open at least a little. Breathing, the beating of your heart, digestion, generating heat—all these things require energy. But the more active you are, the more calories you're burning, and the farther you open the drain to let the energy out.

So here's the simple picture. Water into the sink is consuming calories. Water out of the sink is physical activity. Eat more calories than you burn and the sink begins to fill. Burn more than you eat and the sink empties. The first little bit of energy you store in the sink is sugar—ready to go when you need it. But keep filling it and your body starts to store the extra energy as fat. That's not what you want. On the other hand, burn the same number of calories as you eat and your weight remains stable. And consistently burn *more* calories than you eat, and you'll burn up that stored fat and lose weight. The key, of course, is consistently taking a bit more out of the sink than you put in.

Is the sink too simple?

There are some folks—many with patented diet plans or elixirs, I suspect—who would argue that my model oversimplifies some very complex biochemistry. But in fact it's not a bad representation of your body's energy balance (and a highly regarded principle called the first law of thermodynamics, which recognizes that energy can neither be created nor destroyed). And it has a very simple lesson. But if it's so obvious, why are so many people looking for that magical shortcut to weight loss? People want the pill or supplement that's going to get them skinny with no effort. But the problem is that the most such additives—many of them are stimulants of some sort—boost your energy expenditure artificially and only while you're taking them. They may open the drain a bit, but it's definitely not permanent, and it's probably not very healthful, either.

Are you fat-savvy?

Now that you've learned the Sink Theory, you're ready for a quick true/false quiz on weight gain and loss.

1. Burning fat as a fuel is the key to weight loss.   True/False
2. Running always burns a lot more calories than walking.   True/False
3. Muscle turns to fat when you stop exercising.   True/False
4. Be active enough and you can eat anything you want and not gain weight.   True/False
5. A high-protein/low-carbo diet makes you burn more fat and lose weight.   True/False
Bonus. Low-intensity exercise burns more fat than high-intensity.   True/False

Now check your answers below.

1. Is burning fat the key to weight loss?

False. This is a classic misunderstanding, and I think it was brought about by well-intentioned, thong-clad fitness instructors who urged on their aerobics classes with exhortations to "burn off that fat." As I noted in my discussion of the Sink Theory, your body has two primary stores of energy, fat and carbohydrate (or sugar). Carbos are a better source of quick energy, but your body uses the fats and carbos in different proportions depending on how much energy you're using, how quickly it's needed, and of course what your body has available. But burning one or the other does not appear to make for better long-term weight loss.

Your focus should be on two things: eating a moderate, balanced diet and burning calories. As long as you're opening the drain in the sink—as long as you're burning *any* type of calories—then you're working toward lowering the water level and losing weight. As you get closer to permanently lowering the water level in the sink, you get closer to eliminating some of your stored fat. So don't focus on burning fat for fuel, focus on burning calories—if you do, your body will take care of the fat.

2. Does running always burn a lot more calories than walking?

False. Frankly, which activity you choose does not determine the number of calories you burn—how hard you pursue it does. So running fast burns more calories than jogging slowly (of course, you say), and walking fast burns more than walking slowly (still obvious, right?). But walking fast can burn as many or even more calories than jogging. In fact, bicycling, swimming, and even washing the car vigorously can all burn more calories than running, and that seems counterintuitive to lots of people. The proof is in your heart rate.

How fast your heart is beating during exercise reflects your level of effort and the amount of oxygen your muscles need. Oxygen is a critical component of the calorie-burning process. A higher heart rate means more oxygen and fuel burned. So if a 125-pound woman walks 3 miles in an hour, she might burn 220 calories; if she covers 4 miles in an hour (and therefore increases her heart rate), she'll boost this to 310 calories. Remember, it's all about heart rate, oxygen, and energy expended.

Certainly a very *fast* run will burn more calories than a moderate-paced fitness walk, but here's the real question—do most people really feel ready to head out and sustain a very fast run for 30 minutes? Even more important, how would most feel when it was time to come back and do it tomorrow? And the next day?

That's why walking is such a perfect choice—it lets you start at a reasonable pace and safely increase the speed (and the calorie burn) as you increase in fitness.

3. Does muscle turn to fat when you stop exercising?

Really false. I sometimes hear this as an excuse for not beginning to exercise. "Well, if I get in shape and get muscular and then have to stop exercising, it will all just turn to fat."

Muscle and fat are two entirely different types of tissue, and one cannot turn into the other. Fat is one way the body stores fuel. (Fat also does other things, such as act as padding around joints.) But a muscle is made up of living cells that can never turn into fat. Certainly muscles can become smaller if you stop exercising them, and if you keep eating the same amount of food as when you were exercising you might begin to put on weight and store more fat on your body. So sure, if you stop exercising and keep eating, you might gain fat, but muscle will never actually turn into fat. In fact, muscles burn calories all the time—even when they're not exercising—simply to live. So building muscle is an important part of maintaining a healthy weight.

4. If you're active enough, can you eat anything?

Mostly false. Endurance athletes I've known call this the Hot-Furnace Theory, usually as they're downing a bag of Doritos and a beer. Their idea is that if the fire in the furnace—your body—is hot enough, it will burn calories from any type of fuel. So if you're very active, you don't have to sweat how much (or even what) you eat. For example, if you were to really get into exercise—say, regularly walking 10 miles a day really fast—you could burn 1,000 or more calories in your workouts. That's on top of the calories you need just to stay alive and healthy (perhaps 1,200 to 1,500 a day).

But here's where the Sink (and Furnace) Theories fall short. They don't take into account the fact that your body still has a need for a broad mix of nutrients and fiber. Eating lots of junk won't help it at all. Also, 10 miles a day is an extreme example; in my experience it's pretty rare for people to be active enough in regular daily life to burn such huge numbers of calories. Add to this the fact that if you're trying to *lose* weight, you'd actually like a little daily caloric deficit—you want the drain to be letting out a little more water each day than you put in. Don't use the fact that you're exercising as an excuse to start eating tons of food—especially junk food. Use it as a chance to get to a healthy weight and stay there.

5. Does a high-protein diet make you burn more fat and lose weight?

Really false. You probably know that people have written entire books on this subject. If you eat certain types of foods, they say—specifically more proteins (and, some say, fats) and fewer carbohydrates—then your body is inclined to burn more fat. Unfortunately, most nutritional experts have agreed that this is a pretty unlikely, and especially unhealthy, scenario. Analyses of such diets often show them to simply be calorically restrictive: You eat fewer calories in a day. Some proponents of such diets admit as much, offering that eating fat-laden foods leaves you more satisfied and thus willing to eat less.

But there's a hidden danger here—we know that some types of fat bring risks all their own. For example, the saturated fats and partially hydrogenated fats so common in processed foods are known to help push up your LDL numbers (that's the bad cholesterol). The real point is this: Don't count on any silver bullet or miracle diet. Stick with balanced, healthy nutrition and regular exercise to get to and maintain a healthy weight.

Walk Talk Bonus: Does a slow walk actually burn more fat than a fast walk or run?

False. This was a theory that got the attention of the public a few years back. The basic answer is no. Always remember, it doesn't really matter what fuel your body is burning—fat or carbohydrates. If you generally burn more calories than you eat, you'll lose weight.

The belief that you can somehow burn more fat by doing less comes from the fact that your body does tend to get a greater percentage of its energy from fat when you're less active. But turn up the engines by increasing your physical activity, and your body calls up more fuel. What does it prefer? Easy-to-burn carbohydrates. So if you look only at percentages, it looks like you're burning less fat as you do more work.

That's where people got faked out: What's dropping is the *percentage* of the energy that comes from fat. The actual number of fat calories burned is rising. Even more important, you're burning lots more calories overall, and that's what matters most of all.

7

Making Food Work for You

Dr. Kelly Brownell, an obesity researcher at Yale University, has called America a toxic environment. Not as in toxic waste; as in a profusion of food that is literally toxic to our systems. Or at least toxic in the quantities that we're eating those foods right now. After all, one order of fast-food french fries won't kill us, but an order a day just might. Brownell's point is that we make high-fat food with low nutritional value so easily available, cheap, and tasty—and we market it so heavily—that it's too easy for Americans to take the path of least resistance and eat the stuff. All the time. And gain lots of weight.

What has the answer been for too many people? Go on a diet. A crash diet, cabbage diet, grapefruit diet, no-sugar diet, low-carbohydrate/high-protein diet, or, in a word, *fad* diet. This is when *diet* is a nasty word. The unifying elements of these diets are generally that:

- They claim to have found the magical secret key to weight loss.
- Using this key will finally make it easy—practically effortless—to lose weight.

Unfortunately, research has shown that there is no magical key. It comes down to this: a *healthy, balanced diet*. To get there, you have to detoxify your environment.

Five rules for healthier eating

Here are five rules for a healthier diet. They don't give specific quantities or calorie counts. If you feel you'd like that kind of detailed guidance, go to a broad-based book on nutrition or (even better) see a registered dietitian or nutritional counselor. Just don't turn to a specific fad diet, and stay away from anything that promises to peel off a certain number of pounds in a certain amount of time. Instead, focus on the general tenets of healthy eating. That's essentially the framework outlined on the U.S. Department of Agriculture's food guide pyramid.

1. Drink more water all the time

In many ways water truly is the elixir of life; it's especially important to an active body. The standard recommendation is to drink eight 8-ounce glasses of water a day. For vigorous activity or hotter conditions, you might even need twice that much.

Note that I'm specifically talking about water here. Not sodas, or energy drinks, or juices. Keep in mind that drinks with caffeine (most carbonated drinks, coffee, and tea) are actually diuretics,

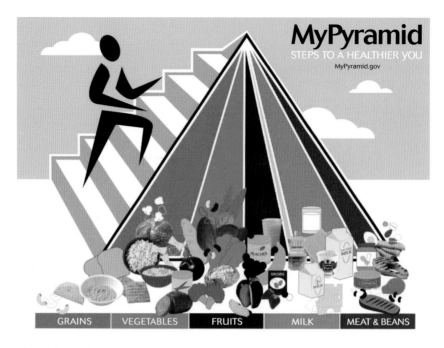

The updated (2005) food guide pyramid outlines a healthy balanced diet, with an increased emphasis on plentiful carbohydrates with whole grain and fiber, lots of fruits and vegetables, low-fat dairy options, and a very moderate intake of high-fat foods.
Source: U.S. Department of Agriculture

which act to dehydrate you; on net, you lose water. Energy drinks contain sugar and calories needed by athletes in endurance competitions. But unless you're charging through two-hour or longer walks, they're probably just excess calories for someone trying to lose weight.

Tips for success:

- Keep a full water bottle at your desk, the car, the kitchen counter, wherever you are, and sip constantly throughout the day.

- During exercise of an hour or more, take water along or know where you're going to stop for it.

- Keep a bottle of cold water in the refrigerator so you'll grab that instead of soda.

- Try carbonated water if you find it more palatable. Just watch out for added sugar.

2. Eat lots more fruits and vegetables

The food guide pyramid recommends at least five serving of fruits and vegetables a day. Many of us fall far short of this goal, but it shouldn't be that hard to hit and even exceed. The key is to think of fruits and veggies not only at mealtime but also for snacks or food on the run. An apple in the car, a banana for dessert, or an orange as an evening snack are all more convenient than fast food or highly processed snacks, and they're vastly better for you.

Also remember that deeply colorful fruits and vegetables are especially nutritious. For example, darker leafy vegetables—spinach, red leaf lettuce—are packed with vitamins compared to their blander counterpart, iceberg lettuce.

Walk Talk: Why is it so important to drink a lot of water?

- Water aids in the digestion and absorption of foods through the intestinal walls.
- Water is important in the elimination of metabolic wastes.
- Our thermoregulatory system depends critically on water. If you don't have enough water to sweat, you can't receive the natural cooling benefit of water evaporating from your skin.
- Most of your blood is water, so being well hydrated is central to maintaining a healthy blood volume. If blood volume drops, the natural cooling process of sending blood to the skin's surface is impaired, and the heart rate is unnaturally elevated.
- Water can be a healthy and natural appetite suppressant. Certainly, drinking water frequently can help give a sense of fullness. But I've also realized that there are times when I'm tempted to eat something cold (such as, say, ice cream) when in fact I'm really just thirsty.

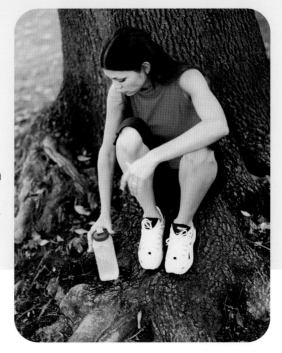

Tips for success:

- Start by keeping a bag of already peeled and cleaned mini carrots in the fridge for snacks.
- Always keep a full bowl of assorted fruits on the counter. Get in the habit of grabbing them for snacks. (It gets easier if you don't keep unhealthy alternatives like chips or other processed snacks in the house.)
- Think about how many colors you've eaten every day. A variety of colors (and I'm not counting cheese curls) suggests a good range of nutrients from fruits and vegetables.

3. Search out whole grains and fiber

Medical research has lately been singing the unabashed praises of dietary fiber (in an academic, medical-journal kind of way). It boils down to the fact that individuals with high fiber diets see improved risk factors for cardiovascular disease, including overweight, blood pressure, and cholesterol levels. That's probably for several reasons. Fiber-laden foods are more filling, so you tend to eat less. Also, fiber tends to slow the rate at which nutrients are absorbed right after a meal, which moderates your insulin levels. Some types of fiber even help keep your arteries clear by lowering your levels of LDL cholesterol.

Tips for success:

- More fruits and vegetables (rule 2) will help. But make a special effort to have fiber in your breads and cereals, too. Sprinkle flax meal on your yogurt for a tasty boost.
- Read the labels for fiber content and ingredients. For example, if you're buying wheat bread, be sure it's made with *whole*-wheat flour, not just enriched wheat flour.
- Seek out breakfast cereals with five or more grams of fiber per serving.

4. Eat fewer bad fats and more good ones

All fats are not created equal. Some are much more unhealthy for our systems than others. It boils down to this: There really are good fats and bad fats. Monounsaturated and polyunsaturated fats—what you'd find in unprocessed vegetable oils, nuts, and fish—may actually help raise HDL (the good cholesterol) levels in your blood. On the other hand, saturated fats—largely found in meat, poultry, and full-fat dairy products—and partially hydrogenated fats are big problems. Hydrogenated fats are also called trans fats; they're created through a process of hardening liquid vegetable oils into semisolids. Saturated and hydrogenated fats are known to both boost LDL levels and increase cardiovascular disease risk.

Tips for success:

- Replace fats with nonfats (or good fats) whenever you can: jam or natural peanut butter instead of full-fat cream cheese on a bagel; mustard instead of mayonnaise on a sandwich; pretzels instead of chips on the side.
- Avoid fast-food french fries, onion rings, and other fried foods, which are usually fried in partially hydrogenated vegetable oils. Cook with olive oil instead of butter.
- Don't use stick margarines; the softer it is at room temperature, the better.
- Read labels, especially on processed foods. Stay away from those with hydrogenated or partially hydrogenated vegetable oils.

KEEP YOUR FATS IN BALANCE
When you're cooking or snacking on foods with fat, focus on the left column and stay away from the right.

More of These	Instead of These
Olive, flaxseed, canola, and nut oils (loaded with poly- and monounsaturates)	Shortening and margarine (usually from hydrogenated oils)
Fish (a great source of omega-3 fatty acids, which boost HDL levels)	Red meat (a source of saturated fats)
Skim or 1 percent milk, nonfat yogurts (great sources of calcium)	Cream, whole milk, and full-fat ice cream (heavy on saturated fat)
Nuts and seeds (in moderate amounts, a great snack)	Chips or other fried or processed snacks
Natural nut spreads (for example, natural peanut butter)	Processed nut butters with partially or fully hydrogenated oils

5. Get more functional foods in your diet

As I write this book, the search for foods with preventive or even healing powers is a hot topic. But don't think it's all bunk—many foods have been well established to be rich in nutrients and to have real disease-preventing power. Yes, food can do more than be fun to eat or simply provide energy. For example, antioxidants (found in lots of fruits and vegetables) may help forestall much of the damage at the cellular level that we attribute to aging, while phytochemicals (for example, in blueberries and plums) are associated with reduced risk of cancer. There are entire books on the health-promoting powers of food. But don't get overwhelmed trying to retool your kitchen. Instead start gradually, making sure you eat familiar healthy foods regularly. Then try out at least one new healthy choice each week; if you like it, make it a regular addition to your shopping list.

FIFTEEN FAMILIAR FOODS YOU SHOULD BE SURE TO EAT

Isn't it nice to know that some of your grandmother's old standbys have proven to be some of the best foods for fighting cancer and heart disease? Here are just a few of the nutritional powerhouses you're likely to find in your kitchen—eat up!

1. **Oatmeal.** High in fiber, famed for reducing heart disease risk
2. **Sweet potatoes.** Antioxidants, mainly beta-carotene, reduce cancer risk; also high in fiber.
3. **Broccoli.** High in calcium, vitamin C, and beta-carotene, and found to reduce both cancer and heart disease risk.
4. **Yogurt.** High calcium levels help keep osteoporosis at bay; probiotics (living bacteria) help maintain a healthful balance of microbes in your digestive tract.
5. **Tomatoes.** Full of lycopene, which is found to reduce cancer risk, particularly that of the prostate.
6. **Cabbage.** High fiber content helps reduce cancer risk.
7. **Blueberries, blackberries, raspberries, strawberries, plums.** Found to have highest antioxidant levels of all fruits; thought to reduce cancer and heart disease risk.
8. **Spinach.** High in beta-carotene and folic acid; believed to reduce both cancer and heart disease risk.
9. **Grapefruit, oranges.** High in vitamin C, an antioxidant that helps combat cancer-causing free radicals; also loaded with fiber.
10. **Brown rice.** Good source of trace minerals and fiber; another cancer and heart disease battler.
11. **Legumes.** High in folic acid, soluble fiber, and compounds called saponins, which lower blood cholesterol levels; help reduce both cancer and heart disease risk.
12. **Onions.** Contain diallyl disulfide, a compound believed to fight cancer.
13. **Garlic.** Its active chemical, allicin, is believed to reduce clotting of blood platelets and risk of heart attack and stroke.
14. **Walnuts, almonds.** Contain mainly monounsaturated fat, which appears to help lower cholesterol levels and fight heart disease. Also rich in vitamin E, fiber, and selenium, an antioxidant. A good snack or great on salads and cooking, in moderation.
15. **Tea, green and black.** A good source of antiaging antioxidants (and a nice way to finish a meal).

The 15 familiar foods on page 77 are all excellent choices, but don't just stick with what you know. Here are some less common but equally healthful and flavorful choices that could spice up your diet:

1. **Arborio rice.** A plump medium- or long-grain rice that cooks to a creamy pastalike texture, probably best known for being the main ingredient in the Italian dish risotto. It's full of B vitamins and iron, and it gives you a healthy dose of complex carbohydrates (just avoid serving it doused with a fatty sauce).

2. **Beets.** Chock-full of B vitamins, including folic acid, a nutrient found to protect against neural tube defects in fetuses and thought to play a role in preventing cervical cancer. A fibrous veggie that also contains a significant amount of beta-carotene.

3. **Black beans.** Research has linked the unassuming bean to cancer prevention, particularly of the breast. Their high fiber content makes black beans a potent weapon against heart disease, diabetes, and high cholesterol as well. As a bonus, they're a rich source of protein, folic acid, thiamine, magnesium, and phosphorous—and are low in fat.

4. **Brussel sprouts.** Like tiny cabbages, they're rich in folic acid and fiber, and also provide a wallop of potassium, a mineral that promotes the proper functioning of nerves and muscles, including the heart. Also a good source of vitamins A and C.

5. **Collard greens.** Dark leafy greens rich in bone-building calcium and in cancer-fighting agents known as phytochemicals. Besides protecting against osteoporosis, these greens are full of fiber and rich in beta-carotene, folic acid, riboflavin, potassium, and magnesium. Also, they contain no fat or cholesterol.

6. **Mangoes.** The rich orange color of this fruit belies its high vitamin A content; it's also a good source of vitamin C. Both aid in the fight against cancer, cataracts, and heart disease. Mangoes also add fiber to the diet.

7. **Polenta.** A food that hails from northern Italy, it's made from cornmeal and typically resembles a cake. This low-fat, high-fiber carbohydrate is high in B vitamins and rich in minerals such as iron, which helps in the production of healthy red blood cells.

8. **Quinoa** (pronounced KEEN-wah). While similar to rice, it's actually a botanical fruit from South America used as a grain in cooking. The small ivory spheres are chock-full of iron, magnesium, and B vitamins, including folic acid. Quinoa also contains more protein—a critical nutrient in tissue growth, repair, and maintenance, and the healthy function of everything from hormones to muscles—than any other grain.

9. **Rutabagas.** These scrappy, bulbous roots don't sound terribly sexy, but don't be fooled. The fleshy yellow interiors offer an abundance of fiber, carotenoids, and phytochemicals, all combatants in the fight against cancer and heart disease. An added plus: They contain niacin, zinc, potassium, and calcium, the mighty mineral of bone strengthening.

10. **Salmon, sardines, mackerel.** These fatty ocean fish "swim" in healthful fish oils, rich in omega-3 fatty acids. These ominous-sounding nutrients actually help lower blood pressure and cholesterol levels and the risk for arthritis. Eat sardine bones and all and you get a mega-fix of calcium, too.

11. **Spaghetti squash.** Named for its spaghetti-like strands, this bright yellow winter squash is a terrific source of beta-carotene and vitamin C, powerful antioxidants, and fiber. For a main course, try it with a low-fat pasta sauce.

12. **Soy products,** including tofu and tempeh. Tempeh is made from whole cooked soybeans infused with a culture and shaped into a dense cake. Soy products have phytoestrogens, known to help fight all sorts of cancer, especially that of the breast and prostate. Soy also can help lower cholesterol levels and alleviate the effects of menopause; try soy milk on your cereal.

Date	Today's Activity Goal(s)	Total Minutes (or √)	Stretch? (√)	Comments, Other Activities? (vigorous chores, sports, other exercise, etc.)	Estimated Miles Walked
Sunday	20, core+				
Monday	40				
Tuesday	20, core				
Wednesday	30				
Thursday	40, core+				
Friday	off				
Saturday	1:00				

Miles this week: ——————

Total miles for the year: ——————

Add shin and ankle strengtheners to your core routine

By now either you're in the habit of doing the core strength routine two or three days a week or you've blown it off entirely. If it's the latter, don't fret—just try to do it whenever you can, and consider every day you do one step closer to a healthy, toned body.

If you do the core strength routine regularly, you should now add two simple moves to it—what I'll call "core+." The straight-knee leg lifts and footsies shown in chapter 9 (see page 100) help strengthen and protect two of your most vulnerable joints, your knees and ankles. Especially as you begin walking or hiking on trails or other irregular terrain, strength around these joints can be very beneficial to avoiding soreness or even injury.

Tip for the week. These are both perfect exercises to do on the floor or in front of the television. If you don't have time to add them to when you do your core routine, try them in the evening, or even right before you climb into bed.

WEEK 18

Date	Today's Activity Goal(s)	Total Minutes (or √)	Stretch? (√)	Comments, Other Activities? (vigorous chores, sports, other exercise, etc.)	Estimated Miles Walked
Sunday	20, core+				
Monday	40				
Tuesday	20, core+				
Wednesday	30				
Thursday	40, core+				
Friday	off				
Saturday	1:10				

Miles this week: _____

Total miles for the year: _____

Set some goals and walk toward them

Setting goals, then rewarding yourself when you meet them, is proven to help you stick with exercise. Of course the trick is keeping the payoffs healthy—forget about hot fudge sundaes. For a week of dedicated walking, luxuriate in a hot bath with your favorite music (or the baseball game) on the radio, and orders to the family to bug off. After a month of consistent walking, splurge on the workout jacket you've coveted. Three months could earn you a visit to a day spa and a massage, or tickets to a concert or basketball game. Use a year of solid exercise to save up for a vacation in your favorite walking destination.

Tip for the week. Talk to the family or a walking partner right now about a payoff at the end of this one-year program. Beginning to plan a hiking getaway in the American West or an inn-to-inn walk in New England, or perhaps a walking tour of the French wine country will be a powerful motivator, even on the toughest days, to get out the door.

Date	Today's Activity Goal(s)	Total Minutes (or √)	Stretch? (√)	Comments, Other Activities? (vigorous chores, sports, other exercise, etc.)	Estimated Miles Walked
Sunday	20, core+				
Monday	50				
Tuesday	25, core+				
Wednesday	35				
Thursday	50, core				
Friday	off				
Saturday	50 on trail				

Miles this week: _____

Total miles for the year: _____

Head for the trail whenever you have time

Now, as you're boosting the length of your walks to increase the calorie burn and help with weight loss and control, the program often recommends somewhat longer weekend walks. Over the next 16 weeks, a few walks will even exceed two hours. But rather than fret at the length, get excited about the prospects—these walks will not only build strength and endurance and consume lots of calories, but also open the door to hiking in far more interesting places.

Tip for the week. Put some effort into finding local conservation land, state parks, and trails in your area (see "Hiking" in the resource list at the end of this book). You can use them for walking whenever you'd like, but they're especially good for the weekend walks designated "on trail." Walking on trails will help you build the experience and fitness for walking on rougher terrain, which will make a longer hike a lot more enjoyable.

	Date	Today's Activity Goal(s)	Total Minutes (or √)	Stretch? (√)	Comments, Other Activities? (vigorous chores, sports, other exercise, etc.)	Estimated Miles Walked
Sunday		20, core+				
Monday		50				
Tuesday		20, core+				
Wednesday		35				
Thursday		40, core+				
Friday		off				
Saturday		1:15				

Miles this week: _____

Total miles for the year: _____

You're following the longer, stronger, faster principle

Your program now has the variety and distance to provide the full benefits of the longer, stronger, faster approach to reaching and maintaining a healthy weight. You're regularly walking 45 minutes to an hour (or longer) several days a week. You're building strength with the core exercises, plus occasionally walking on trails. Now it's time to consciously pick up the pace on the two shortest walks of the week (for example, Sunday and Tuesday this week).

Tip for the week. Boost your walking speed by focusing on quicker steps. (Not *shorter* steps— your stride will naturally lengthen as you speed up—but *faster* steps.) Count your steps for a minute and check your speed here; for more details, see chapter 8.

Steps per Minute	Approximate Speed
115 to 120	3 mph
135 to 140	4 mph
160+	5 mph

	Date	Today's Activity Goal(s)	Total Minutes (or √)	Stretch? (√)	Comments, Other Activities? (vigorous chores, sports, other exercise, etc.)	Estimated Miles Walked
Sunday		20, core+				
Monday		55				
Tuesday		25, core+				
Wednesday		40				
Thursday		50, core+				
Friday		off				
Saturday		1:00 on trail				

Miles this week: _____

Total miles for the year: _____

Invest in hiking shoes

It's time to buy a pair of good hiking shoes and start using them any time you walk on trails rather than sidewalks. Especially if you've been wearing athletic shoes, it's time to find more rugged footwear that matches the type of hike you'd like to take in week 32. Look for high-top boots with plenty of ankle support if you'll be on rugged terrain, or low-cut hiking shoes for a well-graded trail. See the tips at the end of chapter 11 ("Is It the Same for Hiking Boots?"), check outdoor stores, and see "Footwear, Rugged" in the resource list to start your search.

Tip for the week. **Get in the habit of carrying (and frequently drinking) water on your trail walks. Water will be the most important and heaviest thing you bring on these longer walks, so start getting used to it. (See "Hydration Systems" in the resource list for creative ways to carry it while walking.)**

	Date	Today's Activity Goal(s)	Total Minutes (or √)	Stretch? (√)	Comments, Other Activities? (vigorous chores, sports, other exercise, etc.)	Estimated Miles Walked
Sunday		20, upper				
Monday		55				
Tuesday		20, lower				
Wednesday		40				
Thursday		45, upper				
Friday		off				
Saturday		1:20				

Miles this week: _____

Total miles for the year: _____

Switch your strength-training routine

If your body becomes too used to an exercise routine, the exercises begin to have less of a strength-inducing effect. Overly familiar weights and movements no longer stress your muscles enough to make them respond. So it's time to update your strength routine by beginning to do the upper- and lower-body routines shown in chapter 10 (see page 115). They're only five exercises each, and once they're familiar you'll do them in less than 20 minutes. Begin alternating them on the three days you currently do strength work.

Tip for the week. Invest in (or find in the house) hardware to make these exercise routines easy to do at home. You'll want:

- **A set of simple dumbbells (for example, 3, 5, 8, 10, and 15 pounds are common).**
- **An exercise mat for the floor.**
- **A solid, flat bench that can safely hold your full body weight.**

Date	Today's Activity Goal(s)	Total Minutes (or √)	Stretch? (√)	Comments, Other Activities? (vigorous chores, sports, other exercise, etc.)	Estimated Miles Walked
Sunday	20, lower				
Monday	55				
Tuesday	20, upper				
Wednesday	40				
Thursday	45, lower				
Friday	off				
Saturday	1:30				

Miles this week: ————

Total miles for the year: ————

Keep up the knee and ankle exercises

As you're building toward a hike in week 32, you should be continuing the straight-knee leg lifts and footsies (from chapter 9) as part of your strength-training routine. Walking downhill can be as hard or harder on your knees than walking uphill, and the uneven terrain of the trail is a common cause of sprained ankles. Add leg lifts to the upper-body routine and footsies to the lower-body routine and you'll add just a minute to each and complement the existing exercises nicely.

Tip for the week. If you're finding yourself especially unsteady walking on trails, consider investing in walking poles. They are usually called trekking or Nordic walking poles, and are similar to ski poles. Some models are promoted simply as workout boosters for walking on level ground. But it's not uncommon to see serious hikers, especially when they're carrying heavy packs on rough or icy ground, using one or two ski poles as balance and support aids. (See "Poles" in the resource list.)

Date	Today's Activity Goal(s)	Total Minutes (or √)	Stretch? (√)	Comments, Other Activities? (vigorous chores, sports, other exercise, etc.)	Estimated Miles Walked
Sunday	20, upper				
Monday	60				
Tuesday	25, lower				
Wednesday	40				
Thursday	50, upper				
Friday	off				
Saturday	1:15 on trail				

Miles this week: _____

Total miles for the year: _____

Hey, how much do you weigh? Who cares?

Have you noticed that the program makes almost no mention of weighing yourself, even though that's a central goal in this section of the book and program? That's because walking just to lose weight can be a very frustrating experience. If the needle on the scale isn't moving fast enough (or at all), you may think you're not progressing, even though you may be burning fat (a fairly light substance) and replacing it with muscle (a heavier, healthy, and calorie-burning tissue). On the other hand, training for a day hike—now that's something worth really focusing on.

Tip for the week. **If you want a meaningful gauge of your progress, repeat the measurements you made when checking your metabolic fitness in chapter 2 (see page 14). If you've been diligent about the program, your blood pressure, cholesterol and glucose levels, body mass index, and even some body girth measurements will probably show real progress.**

8

Burn More Calories: Longer, Stronger, and Faster

Moving up the pyramid

Exercise combined with a healthy diet is the key to reaching and, especially, maintaining a healthy weight. But that leads to the inevitable question: How much is enough? The simple answer is that it's time to take the next step up the activity pyramid.

You should begin exercising, of course, at the base of the pyramid, targeting the surgeon general's recommendation of walking at least 30 minutes a day, plus stretching regularly. But if you really want to turn things around—not just minimize your weight gain, but really start dropping pounds—then you've got to do more. The "more" consists of three main things:

1. **Longer.** Taking longer walks will burn more calories during your workouts and immediately afterward. The warm and flushed feeling that can last for minutes or even hours after vigorous exercise is proof of the post-exercise energy burn that comes with longer efforts.

2. **Faster.** When you can't take a longer walk, it will help to consciously boost the speed of your shorter outings. A challenging but still comfortable pace packs more calorie burn (and fitness benefit) into less time.

3. **Stronger.** Strength training builds both the power and amount of muscle that you carry. This in turn increases your demand for energy all the time, not just when exercising. The result is that your body becomes a better calorie burner even when you're just sitting around.

Of course, all this requires that you invest more time and effort, but you'll also receive greater benefits. Fortunately, it's not a daunting investment—it requires an additional 15 to 30 minutes of walking four days a week, for a total of 45 to 60 minutes on those days. You'll also have to commit to the equivalent of a modest strength-training routine two days a week. I say "equivalent of" because if you think it might be tough to come up with the 30 to 40 minutes for the full routine twice a week, you can easily break the routine into shorter 15- to 20-minute workouts four times a week.

To summarize, to gain both health *and* weight loss benefits, your weekly goals should be:

- Four walks of at least 45—and whenever possible 60—minutes.
- When you have time, a walk that's even longer—eventually two hours and beyond.
- Two or three walks of 30 minutes.
- Two or three days a weeks of strength training.
- A simple stretching routine, at least five days a week.

A young French teacher who loves walking, Kristen has always struggled with her weight. Although she felt she should walk more to lose more, she found it tough to find the time with a beginning teacher's schedule and her daily commute in traffic-choked Atlanta.

The Turning Point

One day Kristen's car broke down, so she made a bold decision to walk the 6 miles home from work that day. Even though everyone told her she was crazy, and even though she was wearing the wrong kind of shoes and carrying bags over her shoulders, she did it! And she vowed to continue walking home from work every day.

A Week in Her Life

Since that first long walk home, Kristen's gotten the right gear and is now a seasoned walking pro. Monday through Thursday mornings she takes the bus to work. On these four afternoons she loads up her backpack, dons her walking shoes and clothes, and walks home. And seeing as how she and her husband have actually moved farther from work, she now gets in an 8-mile walk. On Friday she gets a ride both ways and replenishes her supply of exercise clothes for the next week of walking.

Her Biggest Accomplishment

Proving the folks who thought she couldn't do it wrong.

How Fast Is She, Anyway?

One day Kristen's husband came to pick her up as a surprise, but just missed her. He then spent several miles in stop-and-go traffic trying to catch up with her—often seeing her only blocks away—as she kept up her steady pace.

Her Key to Success

Getting the right gear and making walking part of her daily routine has made Kristen an impressively dedicated 32-mile-a-week walker.

What's Next?

Weight training several days a week with some of the coaches at school.

Shorter and faster versus longer and slower

This is always presented as if it's a choice—"Mark, should I do shorter faster walks, or longer slower ones?" Which leads to the response, "What about long fast walks—or short slow ones, for that matter?" But I do understand the gist of the question: You've got only so much effort to give to a walk, and you know realistically that when you walk for a longer time, you aren't able to maintain as fast a pace. So what should your goal be—to go as fast as you can maintain for a shorter time, or ease back a bit on the pace and manage a longer walk? The answer is: both.

Once you've mastered the habit of daily 30-minute walks, more or less, the next best thing you can do is add to the duration of your walks. It's easy to do and doesn't require any special skill—just gradually extend from a 40- to a 45- to a 50- to a 55-minute walk, for example. (That's what happens in the weekly programs in this book.) Done gradually, it's absolutely no shock to your system, yet over time you can double the calories you expend in a walk simply by bumping up from a 30- to a 60-minute effort now and then. At a comfortably brisk pace, that could burn as many as 400 calories in an hour.

But you may not have 60 minutes to walk every day. Nor is it ideal to always do the same thing day in and day out, anyway. Some days are a bit longer, some a bit shorter, for several reasons:

• Alternating longer and shorter walks gives you mental variety, and encourages you to vary your routes.

• Different-length walks allow you to adjust the workouts to fit your schedule: shorter on busy days, longer when you have more time.

• Mixing up the lengths can improve the impact of the workouts—a longer walk one day and a shorter the next allows your body to rebuild and improve the systems you taxed on the longer walk. On an easier day, for example, muscles are repaired, more fuel is stowed in the cells (hopefully some of it's taken from your fat stores), and red blood cells are built, all in response to your more challenging efforts.

Walk Talk: I live in Las Vegas, and it gets hot during the summer. I don't like gyms and I don't like treadmills. What can I do to maintain a walking regimen when temperatures hit 105 and above?

Like this walker, I prefer to brave the elements before battling the boredom of indoor exercise. If you're healthy and don't have respiratory problems (they can be aggravated by hot and smoggy conditions), these tips should help when walking through the hottest weather:

• **Acclimate.** Shorten and slow your walks while your body gets better at producing sweat and cooling itself naturally, a two- to four-week process.

• **Adjust.** Try for early-morning or late-evening walks and find naturally shaded areas away from large expanses of heat-absorbing concrete and asphalt. Natural-surface trails around bodies of water are especially nice.

• **Hydrate.** Drink at least eight 8-ounce glasses of water a day to stay generally well hydrated, plus at least another 8 ounces every 15 minutes while exercising. This means you should carry water on your walks if needed—and never pass up a chance to drink (water, that is).

• **Protect.** Wear light, reflective clothing, a broad-brimmed hat, and sunscreen on any exposed skin. All help protect your skin and keep your temperature down.

• **Accommodate.** Realize you may have to split up your walks or simply go slower on the hottest days of the year, but don't use this as an excuse not to walk.

Finally, remember that if conditions become bad enough (say, ozone alerts from health authorities), one or two days of walking in an air-conditioned mall or on a health club treadmill may be the judicious choice. One option is to try to find a club or YMCA that will sell you a day pass for those few occasions, rather than require you to get a full membership.

The last reason may be the most important. A physiologist might call it an "adaptive stress response," but in English we call it getting in better shape. It involves tearing yourself down with a physical stress—what we call exercise—then allowing the body to rebuild afterward. Varying the length of your walks from day to day accommodates that process very nicely.

Longer walks have another benefit. Beyond being a great way to burn more calories and build endurance, they are also amazingly soothing. The emotional benefit of a long walk is matched by few other things in this world. Walking is such a natural and rhythmic motion that it's very easy to get into a groove, cruising along at a brisk but utterly sustainable tempo, enjoying your surroundings, and not even noting the passage of time. In the harried world we live in, such an emotional break is like a gift—especially when you can give yourself the gift of an entire hour.

The secret weapon:
picking up the pace

It's not realistic to keep increasing the length of your walks indefinitely. Sure, if you started with modest 30-minute-per-day walks, there's plenty of room to boost your walking mileage quite a bit, at least a few days of the week. But there are only so many minutes in a week that you can devote to exercise. Picking up the pace is the obvious choice for keeping the caloric furnace turned up.

Walking faster: more calories, less time

Faster walks are a great way to get more out of the time you invest in exercise: more bang for your buck. You burn a lot more calories as you increase your walking speed—especially as you push up to 4.5 miles per hour and beyond. That's when walking starts to become inefficient. The human body is well designed for walking at speed of 3 to 4 miles per hour, and most people are pretty comfortable walking at those speeds. But up toward 4.5 miles per hour and beyond, many people find it more of a workout; some even feel the urge to break into a run.

For someone trying to walk off weight, that's actually good news. The more challenging your walk is, the more calories you're burning. But short of taking all your walks on a track or premeasured course, or asking your spouse to follow you in the car, calculating your walking speed can be a bit confounding. How can you be sure you're busting into that calorie-burning range?

First, remember that speed isn't the best measure of your workout intensity—your heart rate is. Someone who's really fit might find walking 4 miles per hour easy, while a beginner might work hard at 3.5 miles per hour. Only if your heart rate is elevated somewhat do you know that you're really churning through the calories. Experts will tell you that you have to reach 65 to 70 percent of your body's maximum heart rate to substantially improve your fitness and burn serious calories. Using a heart-rate monitor, or stopping to take your own heart rate, is the only way you'll know that with certainty. (See page 161 on taking your heart rate.)

Another good indicator is simply how hard it feels. The Rate of Perceived Exertion, or RPE, is a sound reflection of your effort. (See chapter 12 for more on RPE.) An easy way to estimate your RPE is to take the talk test: If you can talk when necessary but you'd find it hard to maintain nonstop conversation, then you're walking at a challenging but safe speed. It may seem simplistic, but it's a very good indicator that you've elevated your heart rate and your body's demand for oxygen while still being at a safe, maintainable level of effort. This should be your goal for at least your shorter walks—noticeable breathing, but not gasping or wheezing.

Quick steps are the key

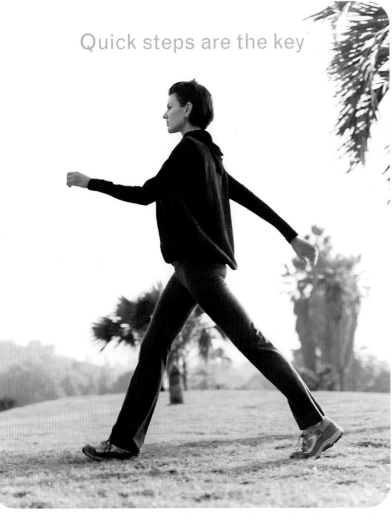

As you boost your walking speed to a slightly higher level, there are two technique tips you should focus on:

1. Maintain a tall posture and relaxed, natural stride. This is the basis of a healthy walking technique, whatever the speed. Remember to keep your head up and abdominal muscles gently contracted, to avoid excessive sway in your lower back.

2. Focus on taking faster steps, not longer steps. As you speed up, your stride will naturally get longer. But that's not the most important thing—taking quicker steps should be your goal.

Some self-proclaimed celebrity fitness experts over the years have recommended reaching for a longer stride as you speed up, but that actually can add to the strain on your lower back, buttocks, and hamstrings (the muscles at the back of the upper leg). Also, if you reach too far with each step, you can actually slow yourself down.

Realize that I'm not telling you to take shorter and faster steps—your stride does lengthen as you pick up speed. Just don't *force* it to be longer. One warning that you're overstriding is that you'll feel a noticeable thunk every time your heel hits the ground. A good quick stride should feel smooth as your heel strikes the ground and your weight transfers smoothly from the foot that's behind you to the one that's in front.

Walk Talk: How do I know if my stride is too long?

Stand with both feet together, as if at a starting line. Now lean forward from the ankles, keeping your body straight like a board, from ears to ankles. As soon as you feel the urge, put one foot forward to catch yourself. Don't try to hold back—just as soon as you're naturally inclined to do so, step forward with one foot to stop your fall.

This is a very rough estimate of your natural stride length at a moderate speed. As you speed up, it will be longer, but this gives you a sense of the feeling your stride should have—not lunging forward for each step, but falling into each step. This is because walking is a series of small falls forward, as you shift weight from one leg to the other. Therefore, it's most natural and efficient to place your foot more underneath your body than way out in front of it.

Figure out how fast you walk

Given that faster steps are related to faster walking, your step rate actually provides a very simple way to roughly estimate your walking speed. It's not as accurate as timing yourself on a track or accurately marked pathway, but it will give a decent estimate based on averaged data. More important, it gives a nice repeatable way to compare your performance on one walk to another. Want to see if you're getting more fit and walking faster? Count your steps at two or three points during your walk. If you're averaging a higher step rate than previous workouts, you can be sure that you're maintaining a higher speed and burning more calories. Counting your steps now and then has another advantage: It simply makes you more conscious of your stride frequency. This alone may help you boost your effort and make your walk a better workout.

Here's how to estimate your walking speed: After you're well warmed up during a walk, count how many steps you take in a minute of walking. A simple shortcut to doing this is to check your watch and count how many steps you take in just 20 seconds, then multiply by 3. (If you're walking especially fast, it may be easier to count just the number of times your right or left foot hits the ground in 10 seconds, then multiply that by 6 for the total number of steps you take in a minute.) You now have your step rate, in steps per minute. Find this figure under the appropriate column for your height in the Step Rate Table and follow it to the right to determine your rough walking speed.

If perchance you do walk on a measured course or track, you can also time yourself for a mile and use this time to estimate your speed in miles per hour, by using the column marked "Time to Walk 1 Mile."

STEP RATE TABLE
Estimate your speed based on steps in a minute

Step Rate (steps/minute)			Time to Walk 1 Mile (min:sec)	Walking Speed (mph)
height less than 5'6"	height 5'6" to 6'	height more than 6'		
100–110	95–105	90–100	30:00	2.0
105–115	100–110	95–105	24:00	2.5
110–120	105–115	100–110	20:00	3.0
120–130	115–125	110–120	17:10	3.5
130–140	125–135	120–130	15:00	4.0
140–150	135–145	130–140	13:20	4.5
155–165	150–160	145–155	12:00	5.0

ESTIMATED CALORIE BURN
For 30 minutes of walking

Speed (mph)	Time to Walk 1 Mile (min:sec)	100 lbs.	125 lbs.	150 lbs.	175 lbs.	200 lbs.	250 lbs.
2.0	30:00	63	80	95	110	126	158
2.5	24:00	73	92	110	128	147	183
3.0	20:00	86	108	129	151	172	215
3.5	17:10	103	128	154	180	205	257
4.0	15:00	125	156	187	218	250	311
4.5	13:20	154	193	231	270	308	385
5.0	12:00	196	245	293	342	391	490

Figure out how many calories you burn

The number of calories you burn during exercise depends on a lot of things—how hard you're working, your fitness level and individual physiology, your body weight (how much mass you have to move), even outdoor conditions such as wind or cold. As a result, standard estimates of the calories you burn during exercise can vary from okay to pretty crummy, depending on how many factors are taken into account. For example, fitness center machines (such as treadmills or stair climbers) that give calorie estimates without even taking your weight into account are typically quite inaccurate. On the other hand, estimates that consider your weight and heart rate (some heart-rate monitors do this) can be reasonably good. But in any case you shouldn't become fixated on specific numbers—after all, you're not going to use the fact that the treadmill said you burned 250 calories on your walk this morning as license to wolf down an extra doughnut at breakfast. Are you?

Calorie estimates that are arrived at by different means really can't be compared. But if you use a standard method—say, a pedometer or heart-rate monitor—you can at least compare the estimate from one workout to the next to see how you're doing. Using the walking speed you've estimated based on your step rate, you can use the table above to estimate the calories you burn while walking for 30 minutes; use the weight column that's closest to yours, or estimate between the two closest values. Keep in mind that these values are for a walk over level ground in normal weather conditions; a hilly walk or a very windy day could boost your effort substantially.

Walk Talk: Is it true that a taller person can walk faster than a shorter one simply because the tall person has longer legs?

This is one of the most persistent explanations I hear of why two people can't walk together. A wife will say about her husband, or a shorter brother will complain about a taller one, "Well, I can't walk with him, because my legs are so much shorter I have to walk faster to go the same speed." Once and for all, forget it—the excuse holds no water.

Your walking speed depends on two things: the length of your stride and the speed of your steps. If you take longer strides (at a given number of steps per minute), then you cover more ground and thus walk faster. Advantage to the long-legged person; the longer your legs, the longer your natural stride will be.

But if you can take faster steps—more steps each minute—then you can also walk faster. That's simply another way to cover more ground in a given amount of time. And the advantage here goes to the . . . *shorter* person. That's because someone with shorter legs has less of a pendulum (that's all the leg is, really) to swing forward on each step. If you expend less energy swinging your leg forward on each stride, you can take faster steps with less effort.

This suggests that these are balancing effects—that the tall walker has a stride *length* advantage, but a shorter person has a stride *rate* advantage. But this misses a key point: There's a physical limit to how long your stride can become. You can increase the length of your stride only a certain amount until it becomes absurd—almost impossible to pull your back leg forward for the next step. But there's no such clear limit to stride rate. As you become fitter and fitter, you can make your steps faster and faster. In fact, world-class racewalkers moving at seven minutes per mile and faster (that's more than 8.5 miles per hour) maintain well over 200 steps per minute for 12 miles! Which is one reason that shorter people are often very successful at the highest levels of competition. At elite levels it's even been suggested that having a long torso and short legs for your height is an advantage—less leg to swing forward on every step.

I'm not aware that this has been proven, but I'm sure that if a shorter person is walking with a taller one, the shorter person shouldn't be trying to extend his stride to equal his partner's. His focus should be on taking faster steps—and making his partner try to match this instead.

9

Going Longer: On the Trail of Weight Loss

Let your walks take you there

One advantage of taking your walking to the next level for improved fitness and weight loss is that it opens a whole new world of walking possibilities. The pessimist might say, "Gee, where am I going to find time to walk for an hour or two or even more on the weekends?" The optimist, on the other hand, is already asking, "I wonder where I can go on

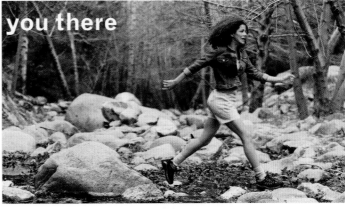

these wonderful long weekend walks?" As you can imagine, the second attitude is much more likely to set you up for success. It's also going to be a lot more fun.

Taking your walk off the road and onto a trail is one of the best ways to stretch your walks beyond an hour. I actually consider occasional weekend hikes part of my reward—payoffs for diligently building my health and fitness during my regular daily walks. But there's more to it than that. Walking on a trail actually improves the quality of your workout. There are lots of elements that can make an off-road walk better for you.

- **Hills.** Walking uphill can burn loads more calories than walking on the level. One research study showed that even if you slow down a bit (which is likely as the hill gets steeper), you still boost your workout substantially. Here's an example of the increase in calories you burn as you increase the steepness of an incline, as compared to walking on level ground at 3.5 miles per hour.

	6% incline (slight)	10% incline (noticeable)	15% incline (moderate)	20% incline (steep)
Walking speed	3.5 mph	3.0 mph	2.5 mph	2.0 mph
Increase in energy expended	16%	52%	67%	70%

- **Rough footing.** The more your muscles have to work to maintain your balance, the more calories you burn. Of course, you don't want to walk on terrain so rough that you risk a serious fall. But even the bumps and rocks of a well-graded trail make your leg muscles work a bit more each time you place your foot, and your core muscles flex more to keep you upright and in control. This slight bit of extra work, added to literally thousands of steps in a multiple-mile walk, adds up. For example, you can increase the calories you burn by as much as 30 to 40 percent by walking on a rough surface versus a smooth one (such as sidewalk), even at the same speed. No doubt that's one reason for the wonderful overall fatigue you feel after a day on the trail.

- **Wind.** You can suffer the wind anytime you walk outside, but as you begin to hike and climb hills your exposure becomes greater. Don't gripe; just look at it as more resistance and more of a workout. (It's also why a windbreaker and foul-weather gear are on the list of essentials for your knapsack.)

Walk Talk: How do I pace myself for walking on the trail? Does it require special skills?

How far or fast you hike or whether you climb a specific hill frankly isn't that important on the trail. Enjoying the setting, your hiking partners, and a great sustained workout should be your focus instead. In fact, peak bagging—charging up hills of a certain height just so you can check them off in your guidebook—is a quick way to take all the fun out of hiking. I'm not saying it's bad to set goals. Okay, I'll even admit that I know exactly how many of New Hampshire's "four-thousanders" (peaks over 4,000 feet) or Colorado's "fourteeners" (14,000-foot summits) I've snagged. I hope to do more of them. But I'm happy to hike up hills I've already climbed, or to heights below the sacred 4,000- and 14,000-foot levels. I think you'll find this a more rewarding approach to the trail. Here are some other rules that ought to help keep it fun.

- **Sip water and nibble food frequently.** Drink water every 15 minutes if your walk will last more than an hour; snacks are a must for ventures of two hours or more.
- **Set a moderate tempo, but keep moving consistently.** Stop as often as you need for food and water, but don't dawdle. The tale of the hare and the tortoise is never truer than on the trail. A consistent, moderate pace will cover more ground than hasty bursts followed by long collapses to recover. It'll be more pleasant, too.
- **Look up from the trail often.** Don't just put your nose down and grind; lift your head a lot to see where you're going and back where you've been—you'll probably surprise yourself.
- **In a group, let the slowest walker set the pace.** If that's just too slow for some of you, then break into smaller groups of similar abilities and plan to join up at intervals, say every 45 minutes, for a snack stop. Just don't let someone end up all alone behind the group—it can be no fun, and even dangerous.
- **Set a turn-back time.** Figure out half the total time you're willing to be on the trail, and set that as the time you'll head back. Then here's the tough part: Stick with your time, even if you haven't reached your goal. The peak, waterfall, or view will be there for another hike—your job is to make sure that you are, too.

Prepping your body for off-road

Your day-to-day walking workouts are the most important way to prepare for a weekend trail outing. They build your basic fitness and general walking strength over time. But there are two other things you can and should do to ensure that your day hike will be enjoyable. One is to take a series of successively longer trail walks to gradually build up to the time you expect to be on the trail.

The second is to add two simple preventive exercises to your after-walk stretching routine three days a week. I'll turn first to the gradual buildup.

Walk longer a bit at a time

There's no rocket science to this—just be sure to build up to a long walk in gradual, bite-size chunks. Let's say you've got a four-hour hike planned for an upcoming weekend. Don't tackle it cold turkey based just on daily walks of 30 to 60 minutes. Instead, over the five or six weekends beforehand you should take walks of two, two and a half, and three hours. This helps your body build the endurance and toughness to handle longer walks gradually. These lengthening walks help stimulate the growth of capillaries, the small blood vessels that deliver oxygen-rich blood right to the muscles. They also encourage your body to increase its blood volume so that you have more coursing through your veins, ready to work when you need it.

There are three specific things you can do to be ready for a longer walk than usual. I call them the three Fs: Feet, Fluids, Friction.

1. **Feet.** It's all about toughness. Not mental toughness—gradually building foot toughness. The best way to do this is to wear the shoes you intend to hike in—not your sneakers—during your longer weekend walks, and even during one or two of your longer midweek walks. This breaks in the boots if they need it, but it also gets your feet toughened to the shoes. A hiking shoe is likely to be a bit stiffer than an athletic shoe—that's part of the trade-off for the increased protection from rocks and increased traction that a hiking shoe provides. You can also try using sandals for casual wear—they tend to expose your feet to a bit more grist and can toughen the skin a bit without the risks of walking around barefoot.

2. **Fluids.** The longer your walk, the more critical it is that you plan to take water along. You should be drinking water on any walk of an hour or more (at least eight ounces every 15 minutes), and in very hot conditions even on shorter walks. It's better to drink too much

than too little—you're body has a very natural and familiar way to deal with a bit of excess hydration. Real dehydration can be nothing short of disastrous, particularly if you're somewhat removed from possible help. Get in the habit of drinking water on your longer walks so you become used to it. You can also figure out how you like to carry water: in bottles in a knapsack or waist belt, or possibly in a personal hydration pack. That's a backpack with a fluid reservoir inside and a hose that you can bring right up to your mouth to sip as you walk. (See "Water Hydration Systems" in the resource list at the end of this book.)

3. **Friction.** This may sound too trivial too mention—unless you've experienced 5 miles of chafing from an ill-fitting pack, too-tight shorts, or an irritating seam in the armpit of your shirt. All seem foolish or even laughable until you've been on the trail for two hours, worn some skin raw, and felt the sweat start to seep in. I hope I'm painting a vivid enough picture that you'll heed my twofold advice:

• Try out all your gear and clothing on shorter walks before taking them on a walk of an hour or more. Be especially vigilant about small rubs or irritation.

• Carry a small tube of petroleum jelly, and don't be afraid to use it. Whether it's applied between the toes or the thighs, or where a waistband or shoulder strap rubs, a quick layer of "lube" can make all the difference.

Walk Talk: How do I treat a blister on my foot—pop it, cover it, or ignore it?

Never ignore a blister—that's the best way to make sure that before long, you won't be able to. Instead, treat it carefully and you'll be able to maintain your regular walking routine.

If it's just a hot spot and fluid hasn't collected under the outer layer of skin (a true blister), simply cut a piece of moleskin in a ring and place it so that it surrounds the irritated skin. Then use a Band-Aid to cover the hot spot. This often provides enough protection to keep it from blowing up into a full-fledged blister—but you have to catch it as soon as you feel the irritation.

Once it's truly blistered up, follow these steps:

1. Clean the area with alcohol or another disinfectant.
2. Sterilize a needle with alcohol or, if necessary, a flame (but remember to let it cool before the next step!).
3. Gently puncture the blister near its base, and gently force out as much of the fluid as possible.
4. Leave the blistered skin on—this protects the tender underlying tissue—and cover it with disinfectant and a Band-Aid.
5. If the blister refills, drain and cover it again. At night you can leave the blister uncovered to allow it to dry out.

Treadmill workouts for the trail

The perfect way to build fitness for walking on trails is walking on trails. But that may not always be an option. In fact, you may find that you want to do some endurance building (and serious calorie burning) on a treadmill. Here are some workouts that might help the time pass while you prepare for the trail. (See chapter 5 for more treadmill information.)

• **The trail hike.**

The goal: Toughen thigh and buttock muscles and prepare for hilly terrain.

The workout: Start with 10 minutes of easy walking to warm up. Then visualize yourself on a rugged section of the Appalachian Trail or the Swiss Alps while tackling the treadmill's preset hill programs. Or you can try 2 minutes each at a 4 percent, 7 percent, 10 percent, 7 percent, 4 percent grade. Follow this with 10 minutes on level ground, then repeat the climb. (If you really need to build mileage, add a third climb.) Finish with a comfortable 10-minute cool-down walk. If you're lucky, the whirring of the belt will start to sound like a babbling brook or the wind though the trees. Your total time is 50 minutes.

- **Fartlek** (that's Swedish for "speed play"). Fartlek follows the theme of alternating faster- and slower-paced walking. The shorter the length of your bursts of speed, the faster you should walk—that's when you really get the conditioning effect and burn up energy. The speeds mentioned in the two examples below are just estimates; pick speeds for yourself that you find challenging and that leave you breathing hard after a burst, but never gasping or wheezing for breath.

Television speed: Walk easily for 10 minutes to warm up. Then watch television in front of the treadmill, walking at an easy 3.5 miles per hour. If you like sports, speed up and slow down with the game. For basketball, burst to 4.2 miles per hour whenever your team has the ball. Baseball? Change speed for every new batter. Prefer soap operas? Just walk at a steady 3.8 miles per hour (higher if you can handle it) and burst to 4.5 miles per hour (or more) during every commercial. Walk eight minutes easily to cool down.

Rock and walk: Load a multi-CD player with a variety of your favorites, from classical to hard rock, and hit the "random play" button. (Or make your own mix on a cassette tape.) After a 10-minute warm-up, blaze at 4.5 miles per hour with Led Zeppelin, then recover at 3.5 miles per hour to Pachelbel's Canon, alternating fast and slow for as long as you can. Finish up with five minutes of easy walking.

Walk Talk: Is walking on a treadmill easier than walking on the ground? Does it burn the same number of calories?

Many people assume that because the belt of a treadmill is moved by a motor, walking on one should be a lot easier than walking on the ground. But this overlooks the fact that much of the energy you expend while walking is spent on lifting your feet and putting them down, swinging your legs and arms forward and back, and even using your muscles to simply remain upright. Walking is really a series of little falls forward—you catch yourself on your foot, vault up over your leg, and fall forward again for the next step. So for the most part, you work just about as hard and burn roughly as many calories walking on a treadmill as you do walking on the ground at the same speed.

However, there can be slight differences. Even a pretty good sidewalk or trail usually has surface irregularities: undulations, bumps, and cracks, all of which you unconsciously adjust for as you take each step. Also, no ground is perfectly level—you're usually going up or down a bit of a grade, even if it's imperceptible. Your body adjusts to these tiny differences without your even knowing it, but they all require a little bit of extra muscular effort and a little bit of energy. The rougher the terrain or more irregular the surface, the more energy you expend.

Some experts point out that as a result, as you get more used to walking on the near-ideal surface of a treadmill you do burn marginally fewer calories than walking on the ground. Their answer? They suggest that you walk the same speed on the treadmill as on the ground, but add a 1 percent incline. They feel that this makes up the difference and increases the calorie burn just enough to make walking on a treadmill equal to walking on the ground at the same speed. But as far as I'm concerned, you need to worry about this only if you're on the treadmill all the time and feel it's not giving you enough of a workout.

Two exercises to protect your knees and ankles

Burning shins, twisted ankles, and sore knees are three of the most common complaints of walkers of all sorts, from competitive racewalkers to trail hikers. You're at greatest risk for all of them, and other injuries, when you're trying to boost your walking mileage and heading onto rougher terrain. But with two simple exercises you can begin to strengthen and protect these potential problem areas. For example, one common form of knee pain results from your kneecap tracking incorrectly where the bones of the upper and lower leg meet; balancing the strength of the thigh muscles can help prevent this pain. The first move also toughens your hip flexors, the muscles at the hip that help pull the leg forward and up on every step.

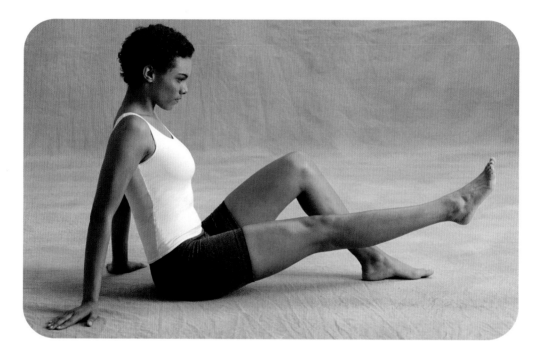

1. **Straight-knee leg lifts.**

• Sit on the ground with your legs straight in front of you. Bend one knee and place that foot on the ground, keeping the other leg straight.

• Contract the thigh muscles of the straight leg so that you see (and feel) your kneecap move, making the knee as straight as possible.

• Lift that foot several inches off the ground and hold for a 5-count, keeping the knee absolutely straight.

• Put the foot down, relax the leg for a second, then repeat the exercise 4 more times. Then switch legs and repeat.

As you get more fit you can gradually work up to 10 repetitions, hold the leg up for longer (up to 10 seconds), and lift the foot up higher.

2. **Footsies** strengthen the foot, ankle, and lower-leg muscles, which get a lot of work on uneven terrain. Sitting on the ground with both legs straight in front of you, forcefully flex the feet into the following four positions, holding each for a 5-count and relaxing momentarily in between. Repeat the cycle 4 times; as you get more fit, work up to 10 cycles.

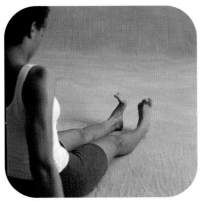

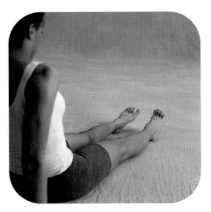

- First, up and in, with your toes pulled up toward you and the soles of your feet toward each other.

- Second, down and out, with your toes away from you and the soles pushed outward.

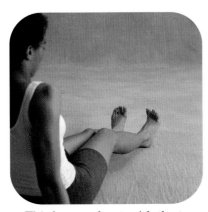

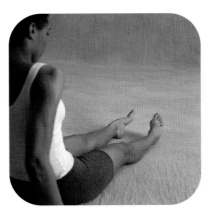

- Third, up and out, with the toes pulled up and the soles pushed outward.

- Fourth, down and in, with the toes pointed away from you and the soles pulled inward.

Gearing up to go on the trail

It seems that whenever I start to lose perspective on how to go about really enjoying a walk in the great outdoors, I have one of those humbling reality checks. One noteworthy occasion came on Windom Peak, a 14,000-foot summit outside Durango, Colorado. A friend and I were sitting proudly atop the summit, having already "doubled" that day—ascended two fourteeners in a single day—with the weather looking like it might hold off and let us snag a third. Ah yes, the sought-after "triple." We'd done quite a job of it, too.

The day before we'd hiked with full backpacking gear 8 miles up Chicago Creek to a magnificent campsite alongside a beaver pond high in the valley. In the morning we'd wolfed a hearty breakfast—well, Pop Tarts and instant oatmeal, but it's just what you need for six hours of hard hiking above 10,000 feet—and headed toward the three 14,000-foot summits. We carried all our foul-weather and emergency gear, plus a full lunch and then some, and kept up a brisk pace. By late morning we were on the second peak and the weather still looked good.

Pretty manly sounding, right? We thought so, too. We were feeling great and hiking faster than all the other groups we'd seen. We had all our fancy gear and were ready for anything, and we were going to bag this triple. So, of course, up trotted a guy in trail running shoes, a T-shirt, shorts, a jacket and waist pack around his hips, and, as far as I could see, one bottle of water.

No hiking boots. No pack chock-full of medical kit, lunch, and emergency rations, no layers of Gore-Tex and fleece, no signal flares and emergency radio with collapsible mini satellite dish antenna. Okay, we didn't have the flares and radio, but we felt like it compared to Mr. Travel-Lite. Who *was* this guy, anyway?

It turned out he was a perfectly normal guy—he just liked to keep it simple. He was superfit, going to do about 19 (nineteen!) miles that day. He'd come in from a distant trailhead to do all three peaks, and would get back out to his car by late afternoon. A few energy bars, hat, gloves, wind jacket and pants, one water bottle, and water-treatment pills was all he figured he needed. He just cruised along and enjoyed the scenery.

Now, I enjoyed the scenery, too, but for a split second I had to envy the simplicity of this fellow's undertaking. No deciding whether he wanted bagels or pita bread with his cheese, or figuring which weight of fleece jacket he'd need. Just get up real early and get walking. Mind you, I'm not advocating foolish negligence in your hiking (for example, he was very experienced and familiar with the area), but it's good to be reminded of three things once in a while:

1. **Don't try to make hiking competitive**. Try to hike farther, faster, or better than the next person and you'll miss more, worry more, and enjoy less. Also, as I've learned many times—there's always someone else going faster, farther, and better than you, anyway. Just ask Robert F. Scott. He's the explorer who reached the South Pole second—by just five weeks. His team perished on the return trip.

2. **Keep it simple.** Have safe margins on food and gear, plan ahead, know your route. But don't make an afternoon hike into an assault on Mount Everest. Hopefully you're out there to have fun and get in some nice exercise, too.

3. **Do it your way.** Figure out what you like about hiking—how far, how fast, what kind of scenery, what kind of company, and what gear works for you—and use this as your guide. Next thing you know *you'll* be the expert, and folks will be asking you what to put in their pack and where to go. (Tell them not to forget the satellite dish.)

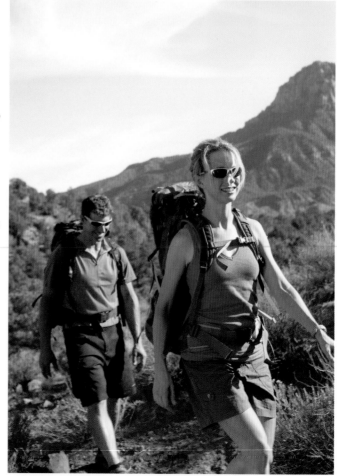

Walk Talk: I've never hiked before.
What should I carry in my knapsack?

If you're really unsure about hiking for the first time, try to tag along with a more experienced friend for your first few outings. Don't know any hikers? Then consider hooking up with an organized group or club (see "Hiking" in the resource list). Most are very relaxed and delighted to have newcomers. They also tend to rate their hikes quite realistically for both length and difficulty, so ask them to help you pick a hike that matches your ability, fitness, and interest.

But you should never count on someone else to take care of you or to have emergency gear for you on the trail. To start, buy or borrow a comfortable knapsack, load it up, and try it out on a 45-minute walk around the neighborhood before hoisting it for a three-hour hike. On top of lunch and any nonessentials you bring, like a camera or binoculars, you should always have the following on any hike that will take you more than 20 minutes from the car. I keep a small bag with the first seven always ready to go—I just quickly check it out before throwing it in my pack. Unique items, such as water purification tablets or map and compass instruction, are available at most outdoor stoors.

1. Water-purification tablets—chlorine-based tablets.
2. Pocketknife. Not a huge one, but a can opener, screwdriver, and scissors often come in handy.
3. Lighter. I usually have an extra stowed in a pocket, too.
4. First-aid kit. Can be small, but it should include aspirin and acetaminophen, several sizes of Band-Aids, disinfectant, small and large Ace bandages, some athletic tape, and safety pins.
5. Whistle. Three loud blasts followed by a break is the universal signal that you're lost or need help.
6. Flashlight and extra batteries. You may not plan on being out in the dark, but it can be a lifesaver getting you back to the car if you're running late. A small light is fine.
7. Compass and map. Be sure the map covers the area well, and learn how to use the compass.
8. Water. Enough for the hike, plus an extra bottle.
9. Food. A full lunch, plus some high-energy food (like energy bars and candy) for emergencies.
10. Adverse-conditions gear for the season. In summer have a hat, sunscreen, and insect repellent. In spring and fall or if you're headed for higher altitudes, always bring a rain jacket, hat and gloves, and extra layers for weather worse than you actually expect.

Layering it on

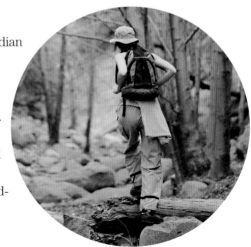

I had the privilege of joining some hikes in the Canadian Rockies with WALKING Magazine readers, and even giving some clinics on walking for fitness, preparing for the trail, and things like that. The night before the first hike I reminded everyone to dress in layers. Even in summer, conditions could change rapidly at those altitudes and latitudes; the temperature could drop 10 degrees in an hour, not counting windchill. With layers, you can easily make adjustments according to the conditions—zip or unzip, remove, and replace as needed.

The next morning as we got ready to hike, I saw several people with layers—all of them cotton. A cotton T-shirt, flannel shirt, and sweatshirt met my "layer" advice, but wouldn't do much good if a drizzle (or heavier rain) accompanied a drop in temperature. Cotton, once wet, has little or no insulating value; it simply gets soaked and keeps you that way. That led to an impromptu strip show of sorts on my part, along with a discussion of proper clothes for layering, following this outline:

1. **The inner layer—next to your skin.**

   The task: Keeping skin comfortable (no chafing) and sweat from building up and causing a chill.

   Good choices: Find wicking fabrics—those that tend to transport moisture from your skin to the outer layer of the material so that it can evaporate readily. Traditionally, silk was the fabric of choice (and it's still the softest feel), but now fabrics like polypropylene and Cool-max (a DuPont material) do the job well. And they're not just for cold weather; their wicking helps sweat evaporate in hot weather, too.

2. **The middle layer—temperature control.**

   The task: Adjustable garments that will offer insulation even if they get damp from the inside (sweat) or out (rain or snow).

   Good choices: Wool is the traditional choice, but polyester fleece materials are the current gold standard. They're light, can be compressed, and come in a tremendous variety of styles and weights to accommodate any needs. They're also widely enough available to be fairly inexpensive. In colder weather you may require more than one fleece garment: say, a lightweight polyester pile turtleneck, then a medium-weight fleece vest or jacket—or, for that matter, a wool sweater. In milder weather a wool shirt or light fleece vest may suffice; in warm months this layer disappears completely.

3. **The outer layer—wind and water resistance.**

   The task: Keeping the wind from sapping your energy, and precipitation from soaking through your layers and chilling your skin.

   Good choices: Traditional outer layers were oil-soaked cotton canvas—surprisingly water-resistant—and nylon and rubberized-nylon jackets. Gore-Tex started a revolution with materials that would allow some amount of sweat, in the form of water vapor, to pass out through them without letting rain come in. Practically every manufacturer now has a material that meets the same standard of breathable water resistance.

   The more challenging the conditions you plan to be in, the more you should go high-tech. For cold, windy, and moderately wet but not soaking conditions, so-called "soft shell" garments are ideal. These stretchable synthetic outer layers offer great breathability and are a favorite for more vigorous activity, such as hiking, climbing, even snowshoeing and cross-country skiing. If you might be exposed to sustained wind and rain, not just passing drizzle, wind/rain pants are well worth the investment, too.

	Date	Today's Activity Goal(s)	Total Minutes (or √)	Stretch? (√)	Comments, Other Activities? (vigorous chores, sports, other exercise, etc.)	Estimated Miles Walked
Sunday		30, lower				
Monday		1:00				
Tuesday		30, upper				
Wednesday		40				
Thursday		1:00, lower				
Friday		off				
Saturday		1:00				

Miles this week: ⎯⎯⎯⎯⎯⎯

Total miles for the year: ⎯⎯⎯⎯⎯⎯

Plan your hiking destination

In week 32 a day hike is recommended as the long Saturday workout. This means your goal should be to get out hiking for several hours—but also to carry food and stop whenever you feel like it to enjoy views, rest, eat lunch, and make it an enjoyable day. Now is the time to start thinking about where you want to go. Will you be most comfortable with an all-afternoon ramble on trails at a nearby state park, or do you want to scale a summit? The more goal-oriented you are, the more you may need to walk to a specific destination like a hilltop, waterfall, or special view. But that's fine—in fact, I think lunching in a special place is part of the fun of hiking.

Tip for the week. How do you pick your destination? Talk to friends, read guidebooks, check Web sites (see "Hiking" in the resource list at the end of this book), and chat up the folks in outdoor stores. Explain your experience and fitness level, and consider bringing an experienced hiker or guide along if you've never ventured into the wild before.

Date	Today's Activity Goal(s)	Total Minutes (or √)	Stretch? (√)	Comments, Other Activities? (vigorous chores, sports, other exercise, etc.)	Estimated Miles Walked
Sunday	30, upper				
Monday	55				
Tuesday	25, lower				
Wednesday	40, upper				
Thursday	50				
Friday	off, lower				
Saturday	1:30 on trail				

Miles this week: _____

Total miles for the year: _____

Add another day of strength training

This week you'll notice I recommend adding another day of strength training a week, for a total of four. To spread them out, I recommend doing the second lower-body routine on Friday, which is normally a day off. The goal is to get in the habit of completing the full routine—upper and lower body—twice a week. In a few weeks I'll simply recommend doing them all at once, twice a week (it will take only about 30 minutes), and you can start doing that now if you prefer.

Tip for the week. Walking on trails encourages stops to eat lunch, take in views, and dabble your toes in streams (all activities I highly recommend). So instead of focusing on your watch, use the pedometer to measure your effort. Here are some very rough step counts you can shoot for on the trail, based on the recommended walking times.

Recommended Time (hours:minutes)	Approximate Steps to Shoot For
1:00	6,000 to 7,000
1:15	7,500 to 8,500
1:30	9,000 to 10,000
1:45	10,500 to 11,500
2:00	12,000 to 13,000

	Date	Today's Activity Goal(s)	Total Minutes (or √)	Stretch? (√)	Comments, Other Activities? (vigorous chores, sports, other exercise, etc.)	Estimated Miles Walked
Sunday		30, upper				
Monday		1:00				
Tuesday		30, lower				
Wednesday		45, upper				
Thursday		55				
Friday		off, lower				
Saturday		1:10				

Miles this week: _____

Total miles for the year: _____

Replace your walking shoes

If you haven't done so since the beginning of this program, it's absolutely time to purchase new athletic walking shoes. You've been walking for six months now, and I generally recommend replacing shoes every three to five months, depending on how hard you are on them and how many miles you log a week. (Another rule of thumb—replace shoes after between 300 and 500 miles of walking.) Check out chapter 11 for tips on shoes to help you with faster walking.

Tips for the week. Pick shoes that will help with the smooth heel-to-toe roll of the walking stride. Look for:
- **A low beveled or rounded heel (not as thick as a running shoe).**
- **Good flexibility through the ball of the foot (and firm support in the arch).**
- **Fairly light, breathable materials in the upper, with no excess layers or support straps.**

	Date	Today's Activity Goal(s)	Total Minutes (or √)	Stretch? (√)	Comments, Other Activities? (vigorous chores, sports, other exercise, etc.)	Estimated Miles Walked
Sunday		30, upper				
Monday		50				
Tuesday		30, lower				
Wednesday		40, upper				
Thursday		45				
Friday		off, lower				
Saturday		45 on trail				

Miles this week: _____

Total miles for the year: _____

Invest in a quality day pack

You'll want to begin carrying some essentials on the trail with you, including water and a small first-aid kit in a fanny pack, but as your hikes get longer you'll need to carry more of these essentials (see chapter 9). So now is a good time to look into finding a high-quality day pack. Talk to experienced hikers and outdoor store staff for guidance, and take your time trying on plenty of styles (the store personnel should be happy to load them up and show you how to adjust them) to ensure a comfortable fit.

Tip for the week. Carry small first-aid kit whenever you're on the trail. Include at least Band-Aids of different sizes, disinfectant, small and large Ace bandages, athletic tape, safety pins, aspirin and acetaminophen, plus your pocketknife. (Outdoor stores also have kits ready to go.)

	Date	Today's Activity Goal(s)	Total Minutes (or √)	Stretch? (√)	Comments, Other Activities? (vigorous chores, sports, other exercise, etc.)	Estimated Miles Walked
Sunday		30, upper				
Monday		1:00				
Tuesday		40, lower				
Wednesday		45, upper				
Thursday		1:00				
Friday		off, lower				
Saturday		1:15				

Miles this week: _____

Total miles for the year: _____

Keep boosting your metabolism

This week includes three walks of an hour or more, plus two shorter walks (30 and 40 minutes) well suited for a faster pace. This combination of longer walks, brisk walks, and your regular stretching and strength training is effectively boosting your metabolism and helping your body become a better calorie burner all the time, not just while walking. Don't stress out if you're not hitting exactly the recommended times. Just keep doing your best to maintain the trends of the program, and you'll keep improving.

Tip for the week. Focus on sound walking technique to pick up the pace on your shorter walks. Think about good tall posture (eyes on the horizon) and quicker steps. If you're not sure you're moving fast enough, consider the "talk test" from chapter 8. Are you walking fast enough to cause noticeable breathing, but still able to speak to (though *not* chat endlessly with) a walking partner?

Date	Today's Activity Goal(s)	Total Minutes (or √)	Stretch? (√)	Comments, Other Activities? (vigorous chores, sports, other exercise, etc.)	Estimated Miles Walked
Sunday	30, upper				
Monday	50				
Tuesday	30, lower				
Wednesday	40, upper				
Thursday	50				
Friday	off, lower				
Saturday	2:00 on trail				

Miles this week: _____

Total miles for the year: _____

Carry all your essentials in your pack

This two-hour walk is an ideal dry run for your day hike coming up in two weeks. Load up your pack with all the essentials listed in chapter 9, carry plenty of water, then hit the trail.

Tips for the week. **Here are some ideas for loading your knapsack for convenience and comfort on a hike:**

- **Place at least one water bottle in an easy-access outer pocket. Pack some quick-energy snacks (raisins, nuts, an orange) there also.**
- **Keep your map or trail guide in an outer pocket, too, but separate from the water so it doesn't get accidentally soaked. Consider a plastic bag (zipper-locking type) for the map.**
- **Place heavy items such as extra water, bulky food, and your first-aid kit lower and closer to your back (and thus more squarely above your hips) inside the pack.**
- **Put bulky but light items like fleece jackets farther from your back.**

	Date	Today's Activity Goal(s)	Total Minutes (or √)	Stretch? (√)	Comments, Other Activities? (vigorous chores, sports, other exercise, etc.)	Estimated Miles Walked
Sunday		30, upper				
Monday		1:00				
Tuesday		45, lower				
Wednesday		40, upper				
Thursday		1:00				
Friday		off, lower				
Saturday		1:30				

Miles this week: ————

Total miles for the year: ————

Fix any problems from last weekend's hike

If you ran into any trouble on your two-hour trail walk last week, don't wait until the night before next week's day hike to remedy the issues. If your boots caused blisters, try new socks or get new boots this week. If you had too little water, get another bottle. If clothing was too hot or cold or itchy, pick replacements and give them a try during one of your walks this week.

Tip for the week. **If you had any physical problems on the hike, it's a good reminder to maintain your preventive habits. Get back to the leg lifts and footsies to strengthen knees and ankles, and be religious about your after-walk stretch routine. This is more important than ever given the stresses that faster, longer, and trail walks put on your body.**

	Date	Today's Activity Goal(s)	Total Minutes (or √)	Stretch? (√)	Comments, Other Activities? (vigorous chores, sports, other exercise, etc.)	Estimated Miles Walked
Sunday		30, upper				
Monday		1:00				
Tuesday		40, lower				
Wednesday		30				
Thursday		40				
Friday		off				
Saturday		Day hike! (2:00+)				

Miles this week: _____

Total miles for the year: _____

Enjoy your hike?

Don't think about time, distance, or how fast you're walking—just get out and enjoy being on the trail. Then answer the following three questions afterward.

1. **How did you feel overall?**
   a) **Great—I was ready to keep going at the end.**
   b) **Fine, but pretty tired at the end.**
   c) **Wiped out. I could barely finish.**
2. **Did anything hurt?**
   a) **Body felt fine the whole way.**
   b) **Fine, but at least one major muscle or joint let me down.**
   c) **I felt like I was falling apart.**
3. **How soon could you go again?**
   a) **Ready to go tomorrow.**
   b) **I'd like to wait till next week.**
   c) **Glad this is the end of this part of the program.**

If your answers were a's (or a's and b's), you're ready to become a seasoned hiker. If you had c's (or b's and c's), you need to build up more gradually and tackle a shorter, less challenging hike—but don't give up on the trail!

10

Getting Stronger

Weight lifting for men *and* women

Here goes a little gender generalization. Men are happy to lift weights to build more muscle—it's socially acceptable, and even attractive for guys to be muscular. Many women, on the other hand, shy away from weight training for fear of bulking up and becoming unattractive; some can be convinced only with arguments that they need to protect their bones from the debilitating effects of osteoporosis. In her book *Strong Women Stay Slim* (Bantam, 1998) Dr. Miriam Nelson, director of the Center for Physical Fitness at Tufts University, recognizes that "Traditionally, women have undervalued muscles. We cared for our breasts, eyes, lately our bones—but muscle's been overlooked." She argues that maintaining good muscle tone is critical to long-term health and to sustaining the body most women want. She's not diminishing the importance of strength training in maintaining healthy bone density; Nelson simply feels that muscle building is just as important as bone building for women. "Many women who think they need to lose five or ten pounds may not need to lose any weight; they often just need to redistribute it, and trade in fat for more muscle," adds Nelson.

As for men, Nelson points out in her more recent book *Strong Women, Strong Bones* (Putnam, 2000) that guys are also at risk for osteoporosis (though not as severely as women); their skeletal health will benefit from strength training and a calcium-rich diet, just as women's will. In a sense, Dr. Nelson points out that men need not look only to hedonism for their weight-lifting motivation, while women ought to!

Weights work at any age

Weight training has been shown to be valuable to adults well into their 70s and beyond. Here are some of the benefits you can expect from strength training at a variety of ages:

- **Twenties and early 30s.** Your body is well suited to building lots of bone density at this age—an investment of immeasurable value throughout your life. Plus, "Muscle is your metabolic engine," says Nelson. Increased muscle mass at this age creates a reservoir of energy-burning tissue for years to come. Nelson adds that strength training reduces the chance of injury from your other sports and activities, and in daily life as well. The stronger and more coordinated you are, the less likely you are to hurt yourself lifting groceries out of the trunk or playing backyard volleyball.

- **Late 30s through menopause.** "At this age it's common to begin losing an average of a third of a pound of muscle per year and gaining the equivalent in fat," warns Nelson. But strength training offers double calorie-burning benefit. During your weight workout you certainly churn through calories. But your increased strength should also enhance your walking speed, meaning your walking workout becomes a better calorie burner, too. For women, muscle is also key to maintaining an attractive, feminine shape. "Women ask if they'll bulk up from lifting," says Nelson, who is adamant that the answer is no. "Stronger is actually more feminine. Fat is loose, jiggly, and bulky, while muscle is trim, firm, and shapely." On top of all her clinical research, Nelson cites the attention given to strength-enhanced figures from Marilyn Monroe to Madonna as evidence of the value of weight training.

- **Fifties and beyond.** Resistance training is credited with maintaining greater mobility and self-reliance, with less chance of injury. " I have people in their 50s, 70s, even 90s hiking, climbing mountains, playing sports. The key is that they've maintained their strength," says Nelson. "The great irony would be to have good cardiovascular fitness late in life, but then lack the strength to be able to go out and enjoy it!" The therapeutic value of strength training shouldn't be overlooked, either. "People with bone or joint ailments like osteoporosis and arthritis may shy away from lifting weights, but they're the ones who will benefit most from maintaining strength and range of motion." Indeed, moderate strength training is often recommended as part of the treatment in some of these cases.

A better build in 20 minutes a day

The goals of this straightforward program are to build basic muscular fitness and control and to help you create a regular habit of weight lifting. Within two months resistance training will be as routine as your regular walks. I designed this program with Donna Richardson, a personal trainer and fitness expert on NBC's *Today* show. She focuses on creating accessible programs that busy women can fit into their daily lives.

For this reason, the workout is split into an upper- and a lower-body routine. You can approach it in one of two ways. Do all the exercises at once and it will take you about 40 minutes; then you need to do it only twice a week.

The other option is do only one routine at a time (it will take just 15 to 20 minutes), but do a routine four days a week. For example, you might do the upper-body routine on Monday and Thursday, and the lower-body on Tuesday and Saturday. Richardson suggests starting this way for the first few weeks to simplify finding time in your day and introduce your muscles to the effort gradually.

However you break it up (two or four days a week), do the exercises in the order given, and do 2 sets of 12 repetitions with only a short break in between, unless stated otherwise. These are introductory movements; they're not complex, and you'll get the hang of them quickly.

- What do I need? The program is presented in terms of using your own body weight, a floor mat, free weights, and a simple bench. With a set of 3- to 15-pound dumbbells, just about anyone can do the program just about anywhere.
- What about the gym? If you go to a club or gym and prefer to use machines, you can simply replicate the moves I describe here. In the more advanced version of the program (see chapter 15), however, I'll specifically recommend using at least some free weights for the balance and coordination that they build.

Upper-body routine

1. Chest press. Lie on your back on a
bench, with weights in your hands and
upper arms in line with your shoulders.
Slowly press your arms all the way out to
fully extended, then back down to the
starting position.

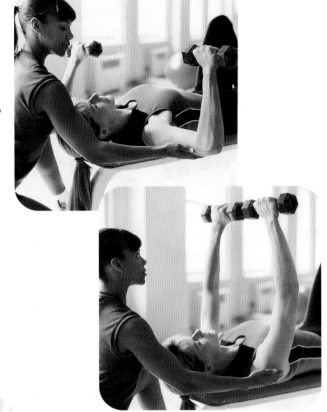

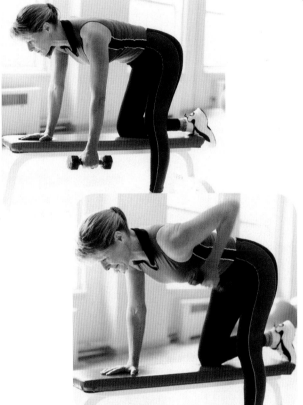

2. Bent-over row. Begin with your right hand
and knee on a bench, left foot on the floor, left
arm hanging down with the weight, back flat
and parallel to ground. Slowly pull the weight
up to your shoulder, squeezing your shoulder
blades to finish; slowly return to the starting
position. Repeat the set on the other side.

3. Abdominal crunch. Lie on your back with your
knees bent, feet on the ground, arms crossed, and
hands on opposite shoulders. Look at the ceiling to
keep your neck relaxed. Slowly contract your abdominal muscles to lift your shoulders off the floor;
hold the crunch for a 2-count; then relax. Start
with 12, but build up to 20 repetitions.

To increase resistance: First, move your hands up
beside your ears, with your elbows out to the sides.
Second, place your feet up on a bench or sofa.

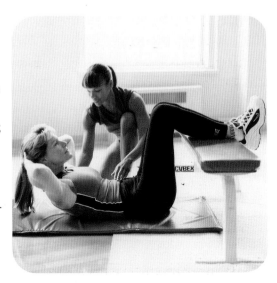

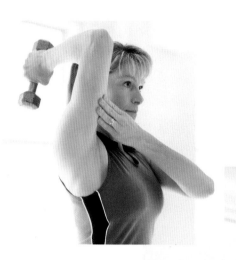

4. Triceps extension. Point the elbow of your right arm toward the ceiling with the elbow bent, forearm down, and hand holding a weight behind your right shoulder. Steady the right elbow with your left hand. Slowly straighten your right arm; fully extend but don't lock the elbow, then return to the starting position. Repeat the set on the other arm.

5. Biceps curl. Seated on a bench with your legs spread, place your right elbow inside the right knee, braced with the left hand. Your right hand holds the weight, and the arm starts straight—slowly bend it until the weight is up at the shoulder, then return to the starting position. Repeat the set on the other arm.

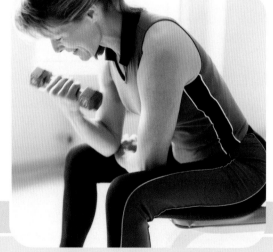

LIFT RIGHT (THEN LEFT)

Here are some tips for effective, safe weight lifting:

- Concentrate on good, slow technique—don't let momentum do the work for you—and move your joints through their full range of motion.
- When possible, exhale while lifting the weight, and inhale on the recovery or between reps.
- Maintain good posture. Focus on stabilizing your body throughout all movements with your abdominal and back muscles.
- Lifting shouldn't hurt, but it should be hard. Select a weight so that you're just able to finish the designated number of repetitions on the last set but would be hard pressed to do more.
- Keep progressing. When a weight becomes easy to lift, add more. Increase to the next weight and reduce the number of repetitions if necessary, until you're able to build up to the full target number again.

Lower-body routine

1. **Abdominal crunch.** Same as upper-body routine.

2. **Lunge.** Start with both feet together. Take a giant step forward while bending your forward knee (maintain a tall posture; don't push your bending knee beyond the foot). Then press forcefully off your forward leg to return to standing. Alternate 10 reps on each leg.

   To increase resistance: Hold light dumbbells.

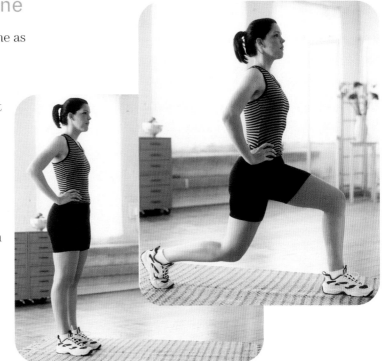

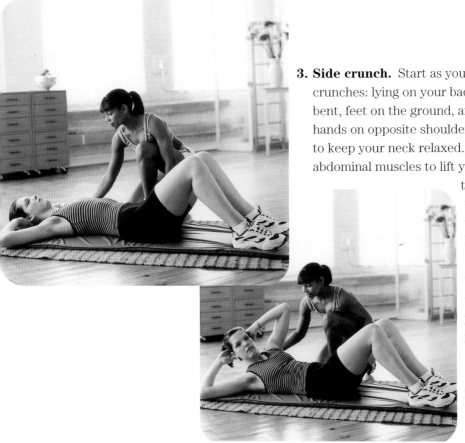

3. **Side crunch.** Start as you did for abdominal crunches: lying on your back with your knees bent, feet on the ground, arms crossed, and hands on opposite shoulders. Look at the ceiling to keep your neck relaxed. Slowly contract your abdominal muscles to lift your right shoulder off the floor, twisting so the right elbow goes toward the left knee. Relax. Do 12 reps in each direction.

   To increase resistance: First, move your hands up beside your ears, with your elbows out to the sides. Second, place your feet up on a bench or sofa.

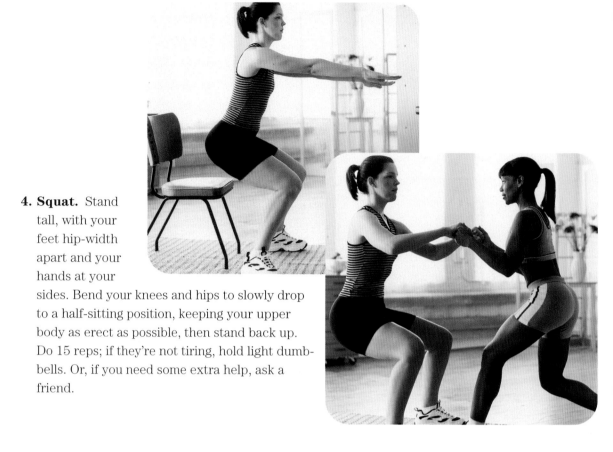

4. Squat. Stand tall, with your feet hip-width apart and your hands at your sides. Bend your knees and hips to slowly drop to a half-sitting position, keeping your upper body as erect as possible, then stand back up. Do 15 reps; if they're not tiring, hold light dumbbells. Or, if you need some extra help, ask a friend.

5. Alternate arm/leg extension. Begin on your hands and knees on the floor, with your head level and your back flat. Extend your right arm and left leg out straight, parallel to the ground. Hold for five seconds, then drop; repeat on the other side. Begin with 6 reps on each side, building to 12.

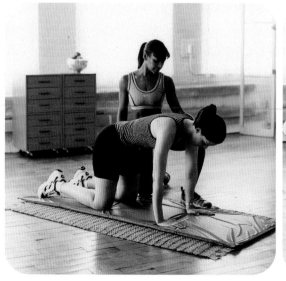
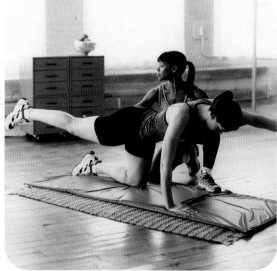

Toys to boost the burn?

The eternal quest to burn more calories in less time drives many people to consider a variety of implements to increase the intensity of their walks. And lots of people want to combine their workouts—why not get in your upper-body strength training while you're walking, after all? But this may be an example of trying to do too much at once—which is why I recommend strength training as a separate activity several days a week.

Some tools for boosting your walking workout sound perfectly reasonable, such as carrying hand weights while walking. Others are a bit offbeat but plausible, like walking with ski poles. And some, like boots with big springs on the bottom that purport to help you bounce your way to fitness—I swear these exist—are downright zany. They may not belong in the Weight-Loss Hall of Shame with the vacuum pants that claim to literally "suck" the cellulite right off your thighs (no kidding—you attach your own vacuum), but don't you wonder who buys these things? Still, a few common walking workout boosters are well worth a mention.

Hand weights

By far the most common supplement to a walking workout, hand weights are marketed widely as an easy way to add an upper-body punch to the cardiovascular workout. Hand-weight promoters will tell you that to get the best workout, you have to bend your elbows and pump your arms vigorously, which is true. They'll also say that you can increase the calories you burn by anywhere from 10 to 50 percent, though independent research suggests that 5 to 20 percent is a more reasonable expectation. What they won't say is that you might get as much as half of this increase in energy expenditure simply by bending your arms 90 degrees and pumping them vigorously—without weights—during a brisk walk.

Also, hand weights bring with them concerns for people who have a history of shoulder or elbow problems or for anyone with heart trouble or high blood pressure. The latter is because the act of gripping the weights can boost your blood pressure artificially, an effect called the pressor response.

Hand-Weight Road-Test Results

PROS	CONS
You may feel the least self-conscious with these, because the vigorous arm action will be familiar to fast walkers and runners.	As you fatigue, you may want to stop pumping your arms; you must concentrate hard to maintain your speed.
Definitely works the muscles of the upper back, shoulders, and eventually biceps (upper arm).	You must speak to your doctor before using hand weights if you have heart problems or high blood pressure.
The weights are ideal for a simple postwalk upper-body exercise routine.	Hand weights could aggravate any preexisting shoulder or elbow problems.

Poling to Fitness: Nordic Walking

Called "Nordic Walking," the idea comes from Nordic skiers who walk, hike, and run with their ski poles in the off-season to keep their upper bodies in shape for when the snow returns. Nordic walking has spread worldwide and as of this writing a number of pole manufacturers are promoting the activity in the US and even training fitness and outdoor instructors in how to teach it. As a certified master coach myself, I now have to disclose a certain bias in support of Nordic walking. But I think it's because I have a full understanding of its benefits. Here's what it does:

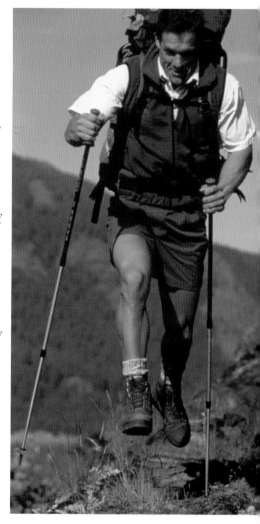

- The movement mimics the stride in Nordic skiing, with the right arm and pole swinging forward with the left foot, and vice versa. Most people find it comes surprisingly naturally.

- Nordic walking adds an upper body workout to walking, recruiting muscles of the arms, shoulders, chest, upper back, lats (those wing muscles under the arms), and even abdominals.

- On average Nordic walking burns about 20 percent more calories than regular walking at the same speed. If you really use your poles vigorously, you can boost the energy expenditure by as much as 45 percent. All this because you're using a bunch of upper body muscles much more than you would in normal walking.

- The poles can reduce the impact forces on the feet, ankles, and knees by bearing some of the load, particularly when walking downhill.

- The poles improve balance on uneven terrain, and can also be an aid to recovery following surgery, stroke, or other gait impairments.

There are a range of poles available for walking, and they *are* different from the ski poles you have in the closet. Four features to consider if you want to give walking poles a try:

1. Hand grip. Ideally it will be ergonomically designed for a comfortable grip.
2. Wrist strap. Very important so that you can pole vigorously without having to clench your grip too hard or incessantly. In fact, as your arm swings forward you should be able to relax your grip entirely.
3. Pole shaft. Some are fixed length, single-shaft poles, others are multipart, adjustable length, telescoping poles. A single shaft offers much lighter weight with great strength, and it won't shorten even during vigorous poling. A telescoping pole is heavier but can be shortened to go in your pack or be adjusted slightly for up or downhill walking.
4. Pole tip. There should be a hardened metal spike tip for good grip on grass, dirt, gravel, and other soft surfaces. But you may also want a removable rubber tip that you can put on for walking on asphalt and pavement; otherwise the metal spike will clatter and slip.

To try Nordic Walking for the first time, use this four step progression. Give it a whirl first on grass so the spiked pole tip will get better "grab" and the poling action is more noticeable.

Step 1: Carry the poles. Grasp each pole at the middle of the shaft and just walk normally, with the poles not even touching the ground while you alternate swinging your arms and legs. Focus on the feeling of arms and legs swinging in opposition—right arm with left leg, left arm with right leg.

Step 2: Drag the poles. Put your hands through the wrist straps, but as you get ready to walk release your pole grips and allow the poles to hang at your sides with only the wrist straps attaching them to your hands. Walk normally, allowing your arms to swing freely forward and let the poles drag behind you, noting their roughly 45-degree backward angle.

Step 3: Plant the poles. As you feel the pole tips poke into the earth begin loosely grabbing the grips in each hand when your arms swing fully forward. Gently grasp the pole and plant it at about a 45-degree angle with the grip forward and the pole tip back. Gently push backward on the ground as you step forward with the opposite foot.

Step 4: Push. Once the motion is comfortable, push backward on the poles more forcefully on each step—this will engage the triceps and latissimus dorsi muscles of the back more completely. Rely more on the strap than the grip when pushing the pole backward into the ground, relaxing your hands and releasing the grip as your arms swing forward.

Give yourself 15 minutes to work through this simple progression, then just go Nordic walking for a while. Most people find they get comfortable with the movement within 30 minutes of starting, though many feel taking at least a little bit of instruction can dramatically improve their technique and the quality of the workout. (For more, see the manufacturers' Web sites under "poles" in the resource list.)

Weight vests

One day I headed out for a walk feeling like a SWAT team member. In fact, I didn't make it out of the office without people asking where my pistol and walkie-talkie were. But I wasn't ready to start walking a beat—just trying out a piece of exercise hardware, a weight vest. There is now a wide range of styles from lighter fabric vests that, with the weights removed, can be thrown in the washer, to heavy-duty plastic models that can carry 30 pounds or more. A lighter front-opening type of vest is probably best for walking. To increase resistance during calisthenics, stair stepping, or other more up-and-down activities, a more rigid vest that's put on over the head may be better.

Research indicates that walking on level ground and carrying 5 to 10 percent of your body weight in a vest increases the calories you burn by only about the same percentage. (Adding more weight than this isn't recommended, because it can cause uncomfortable neck and shoulder strain.) The effect is increased somewhat when walking uphill, since you have to lift the weight against gravity.

The shortcoming of a weight vest is that carrying weight close to your torso is a fairly efficient way to haul a load—backpackers and soldiers learn to put the heaviest items in their packs close to their bodies to benefit from this fact. So if you really want to turn up the heat on a walk, other choices may be better.

My verdict on walking toys

Hand weights, weighted vests, and walking poles are certainly not the first ideas out there for increasing the intensity of a walking workout, and they no doubt will not be the last. Each has its relative merits, but it's important to keep in mind that part of the beauty of walking as an exercise is that, at its most fundamental, you don't need any additional equipment or specialized training. Plus, if your goal is to build some of your walking into your daily life—a trip to the post office or stroll with a neighbor—it's much easier if you don't need a special piece of gear. ("Oh yes, I'd love to join you, Agnes. Hang on a second while I dig out my weight vest. Now where is that thing?")

But each of the three tools here has proven benefits, and hand weights and walking poles provide the added payoff of adding an upper-body workout to walking. The problem with hand weights is that if you add enough weight to really work your upper-body muscles, it could undermine your walking technique or speed. That's why of the three, I give the highest score to Nordic walking. The movement is easy and natural, can provide a substantial increase in exercise intensity, and definitely works the upper-body muscles effectively. It depends, of course, on how vigorous your poling motion is while you walk. Drag them along or place them daintily alongside and they'll do very little for you. But place them firmly with your arm extended (the so-called handshake position) and then push forcefully back on the ground like a Nordic skier, and you'll get a great workout for the entire body.

Walk Talk: Should I consider wearing ankle weights to boost my walking workout?

In a word, no. Research has shown that ankle weights increase energy expenditure by only about 5 to 10 percent—less than you'll get with hand weights. This is probably because your legs are quite strong and the weight is mostly being swung forward and back, not up and down, while hand weights have to be lifted up against gravity with each arm swing.

But the bigger concern is that weights attached to the ankle may cause you to alter your walking mechanics in an unnatural way or—even worse—put your knee joints at some risk. The key variable in increasing your walking speed is increasing the quickness of your steps; adding weight to your ankles will only make this harder to do. It's also been theorized that the added weight could put your knee under strain every time your leg swings forward. Given the fragility of the human knee joint, this is a risk I just wouldn't want to take, especially since there are much better alternatives for boosting the intensity of your walk. So stay away from ankle weights, and focus on quick steps instead.

11

Going Faster: Shoes Matter

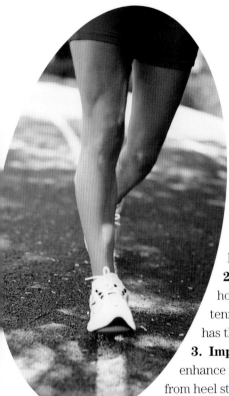

Faster feet need faster footwear

The faster you'll be walking, the more your shoes can help. The quicker stride and rolling gait of faster walking mean your foot will be experiencing a greater range of motion—more flexing and bending with every step. This leads to three simple reasons that any serious walker should be investing in true walking shoes:

1. Fewer injuries. They're designed for the unique heel-to-toe rolling motion of the foot in the walking stride—a stride that's quite distinct from running or other sports. Therefore, you're less likely to suffer discomfort or injury if you walk in walking shoes.

2. Greater durability. A shoe designed for walking is likely to hold up better for walking, just as a tennis shoe will do better on the tennis court, and a running shoe better for running. A walking shoe has the flexibility and support where you need it for walking.

3. Improved performance. A well-designed walking shoe can actually enhance your performance, by allowing a more fluid, rolling walking gait from heel strike to toe off.

Why not a running shoe?

In many stores, if you mention that you're a fairly serious walker, they're likely to try to get you into a running shoe. Even some doctors, fitness experts, and coaches still recommend running shoes to serious walkers. In many cases I think they're hearkening back to their experiences years ago, when the category of "walking shoes" meant walking-around, hanging-out, not-at-all-athletic shoes. Their image may be of stiff, all-white, all-leather nurses' shoes that frankly would be lousy for actually trying to walk fast. This perspective is dated, and unless a physician or specialist is prescribing running shoes for a specific problem or pathology, she's probably wrong.

The best athletic walking shoes now feature materials and manufacturing that compare to the best running shoes—just as durable, just as supportive—but in a design better suited to the walking gait. The design differences boil down to three key factors:

1. Your foot strikes the ground with only one to one and a half times your body weight when you're walking, as opposed to running's much more severe impact—three or four times your body weight. Thus, running shoes need a great deal more cushioning than do walking shoes.

2. In the walking stride your foot generally strikes the ground farther back on the heel, with the toes held higher up in the air, than in the running stride. The foot also rolls from heel to toe much more gradually in walking than in running. Thus a walking shoe should have a lower and more rounded or beveled heel than a running shoe. An extra-thick heel—needed to cushion high-impact running steps—acts only to lever the toes down quickly, which is bad for walking. In fact, a thick, squared-off running heel can even lead to shin discomfort for a brisk walker, because as the toes slap down, the foot pulls on the shin muscles. If your shins burn and you're walking briskly in running shoes, your first step should be to switch to walking shoes right away.

3. A walker rolls farther off the toes at the end of each stride than a runner. So a walking shoe should be more flexible through the ball of the foot than a running shoe. Many running shoes trade flexibility for more padding (for shock absorption) in the front of the foot.

Keep in mind that the more briskly you walk, the more you'll benefit from the lower and more flexible design of a high-performance athletic walking shoe.

Walk Talk: What is pronation, and do I have to worry about it when buying shoes?

Pronation is the natural inward roll of your heel that happens every time your foot strikes the ground. It's one way your foot cushions the impact, and a certain amount of pronation is perfectly normal. But too much (overpronation) can cause shin, knee, and even hip problems; too little (underpronation, or what some people call supination) means you may not get enough natural cushioning on each step.

The best way to know if you over- or underpronate is to have a sports medicine podiatrist check you out; if you're having severe or chronic problems, it's worth a visit. Just be forewarned that a primary tool for treatment is prescription orthotics, those custom-formed soles that go inside your shoes to, among other things, control pronation. Orthotics can be quite expensive, and not everybody needs them—sometimes just getting more appropriate walking shoes can make a big difference.

If you're not having problems, use the simple but less accurate alternative of looking at one of your old pairs of athletic shoes. Set them on a table side by side, and view them from behind. If the heel cups lean in toward each other (because the cushioning material on the inner side of the heel is more compressed), then you probably overpronate. If they lean outward, you probably underpronate. Here's what to look for in shoes, depending on what you find:

- **Overpronators.** Pick walking shoes with all the recommended features, plus look for especially firm material under the inside of the heel. Sometimes it's simply a harder, higher density of foam material (often a different color from the rest of the midsole), but sometimes it's a rigid plastic piece molded right into the sole. It's often called a medial post, so if you really want to sound like a shoe geek, ask for one at the shoe store.
- **Underpronators.** Your goal is to make up for the cushioning motion your feet naturally lack. Look for well-designed walking shoes, but choose models that are especially well cushioned. Try for some of the fairly rare models that have polyurethane (PU) foam in the heel (a slightly heavier but more durable foam than the ethyl vinyl acetate—EVA—that's typically used). Or consider models that carry the manufacturer's best and most durable cushioning technology, such as air, gel, or other high-density foams in the heel.

The twist 'em, bend 'em, poke 'em shoe tests

Three simple tests will help give you a sense of how well a shoe is designed for walking. Do them right in the store with the salespeople watching and maybe they'll learn something, too.

1. **Poke 'em, step 1.** A walking shoe should have a fairly low, rounded or beveled heel. This eases the transition as the heel first strikes the ground, and it allows the foot to roll from heel to toe gradually and smoothly, not abruptly. Push down firmly with a pencil at the very back of the shoe, inside the cup that surrounds the heel. If the heel is rounded or beveled sufficiently, the toes will lift off the ground.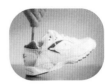

   Step 2. The end of a smooth heel-to-toe roll is aided by a noticeable bend upward at the toe of the shoe, called toe spring. Push down on the end of the toe—the more the heel lifts off the surface, the more toe spring the shoe has. (The faster you walk, the more heel bevel and toe spring you'll appreciate in your shoes.)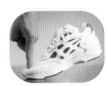

2. **Bend 'em.** At the end of each stride, your foot bends through the ball of your foot just before you toe off. Grab the heel of the shoe firmly and push upward at the toes to see that the shoe bends where your foot naturally does, not under the arch. If the shoe does bend through the arch, stay away; this lack of support can lead to discomfort in the bottom of your foot and arch.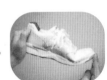

3. **Twist 'em.** As your foot accepts your weight, you imperceptibly load the outside of your foot first (the little toe), then shift your weight inward to the big toe. This slither from little toe to big happens quickly, without your even knowing it, but it's aided by a shoe with a bit of torsional flexibility. Grab the heel and toe of the shoe firmly and give a twist to look for modest flexibility, so your foot's independent suspension can do its work.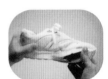

Is it the same for hiking boots?

You have to match the hiking shoes you choose to the conditions you'll be using them in. Strolling on gently graded trails on nearby conservation land doesn't require the same boot as scrambling up a basalt-strewn volcano (dormant, you hope) in western Oregon. But hiking shoes do five basic things, and how much you need of each determines what the shoe looks like.

1. **Protect your foot from sharp and uneven bumps in the trail.** The bottom of a hiking shoe is fairly thick, and has to be firm to protect the bottom of your foot. But the thicker and firmer the sole of the shoe, the more flexibility you sacrifice.
   The trade-off: The rougher the trail and sharper the rocks, the stiffer and thicker the sole should be.

2. **Protect you from twisting your ankle.** The irregularities of hiking trails, let alone scrambling on rocks, can put you at risk for rolling or spraining an ankle. So many styles are high-top boots that protect the ankle. But there are also mid- and low-cut styles designed for more regular terrain and smooth trails.
   The trade-off: More ankle protection means a heavier and warmer shoe (since most heat escapes out the top of the boot).

3. **Protect your foot from scrapes and bruises.** Sharp rocks and rough surfaces, especially when scrambling, can bang up your feet. Your toes are especially vulnerable when you are scrambling uphill. If you'll be on rough and rocky terrain, look for a thick rubber band around and even on top of the toes.

The trade-off: More toe protection means a heavier and hotter boot.

4. **Protect your foot from the elements.** Weatherproof leathers and even Gore-Tex or similar breathable liners are now common in rugged footwear. You pay a lot for the added protection, and despite how breathable many claim to be, in my experience they do tend to make your feet warmer.

The trade-off: Truly waterproof boots are fine in cool, consistently wet conditions, and they're a must for winter hiking and snowshoeing. But they may not be worth the price (and added heat) for hikers concerned only about getting caught in an occasional summer rain or splashing across a creek.

5. **Provide traction.** You don't want to be scrambling up a sloping rock face or descending through loose scree (like gravel) when you realize your boots don't have enough grab. But keep in mind that traction depends on two things: the softness of the rubber on the sole and the depth of the lugs or tread pattern.

Trade-off 1: Softer rubbers are great on slick rocks and regular surfaces, but they tend to wear out more quickly. They're a good choice for the outdoor sandals you'll wear when kayaking, for example, or scrambling the slickrock of Moab, Utah.

Trade-off 2: A deep tread will improve the grab on rough terrain, dirt, and gravel, but it also makes the boot heavier and stiffer. So don't buy more tread than you need.

Walk Talk: How can I be sure my shoes fit?

Before deciding on a specific brand or style of shoe, make sure the pairs you're considering fit properly. Here are a few tips to ensure that your shoes will treat your feet right:

• Wear the socks that you'll normally wear in the shoes, especially if you prefer walking socks with thicker padding in the heel and toe.

• Buy later in the day, or walk around a lot before going in to buy, so that your feet have swelled to full size.

• Always try on both shoes—one foot is often a half to a full size larger than the other.

• Walk on a hard surface when you're trying on the shoes, not just on carpeted floor. And be sure to do some full-speed walking to check for rubbing or irritation.

• If you have a narrow or wide foot, insist on a width-sized shoe. If they don't have any, go to another store. Enough manufacturers offer a wide enough variety of widths that you should be able to find a pair that works for you. (You can also buy online—see "Footwear" in the resource list at the end of this book—but be prepared to send them back if the fit isn't right.)

• *Never* let a sales associate convince you that a shoe will "break in" and feel better. If it doesn't feel right in the store, it won't feel right on the road.

• Don't settle for a shoe that's not quite right. It will only aggravate you and cause you to stop walking.

• If it's a hiking shoe or boot, climb up on the incline surface, or simply jam your feet hard on a carpeted surface, to make sure your toes won't slam into the end of the boot when you walk downhill.

The three key checkpoints for a good fit:

1. Your longest toe should never touch the end of the shoe at any point during a step.
2. Your heel shouldn't slip in and out during a stride.
3. There should be no pinching or binding across the top of the foot, or at the widest part of the foot, especially as your foot flexes at the end of a step.

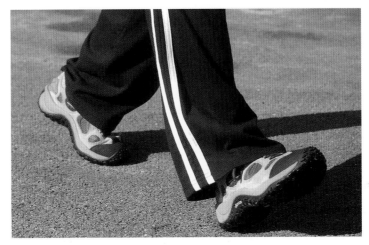

These "rugged walking" shoes have the rounded heel and flexible forefoot for the heel-to-toe walking stride, but added tread and support for the trail.

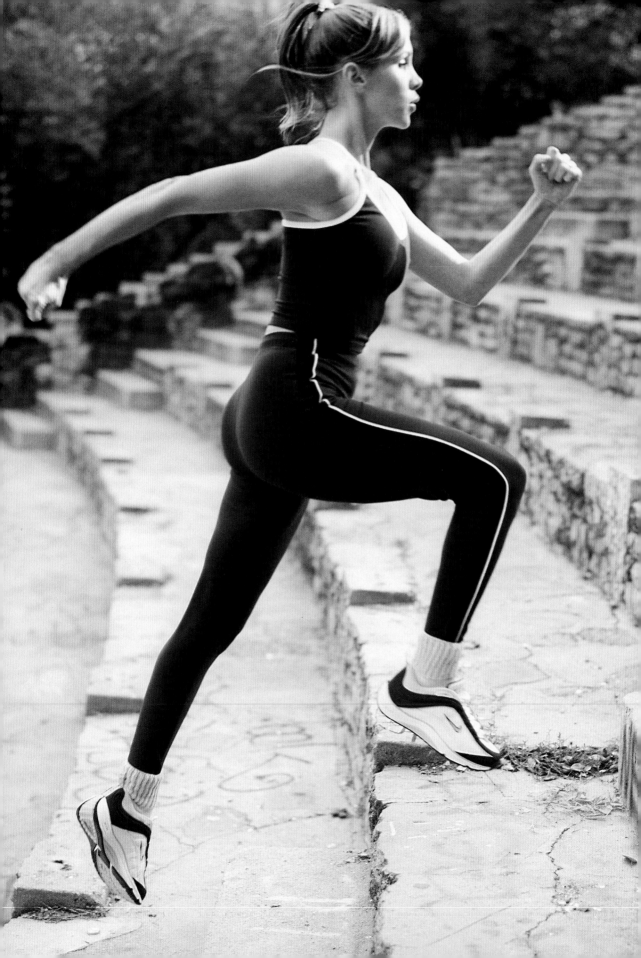

Part III

Getting Fit: Building Speed and Strength

The satisfaction we derive from games is complex. We enjoy struggling to get the best of ourselves. . . . It is not just the desire to succeed. It is the need to feel that our bodies have a skill and energy of their own, apart from the man-made machines they drive.

ROGER BANNISTER
THE FOUR-MINUTE MILE, 1955

12

Finding the Athlete Within

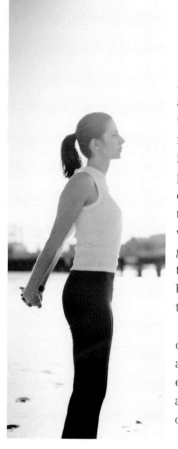

A couple of years ago I had the opportunity to teach a fellow editor at *WALKING* Magazine how to racewalk. The idea was that she'd then be able to give a firsthand account of the virtues and glories of racewalking to the readers of the magazine. Unfortunately, to make it more realistic, the task of guinea pig/journalist fell to a self-proclaimed athletic late bloomer, Ann. To say that Ann wasn't into competitive sports would be to say that Wimbledon is just another tennis tournament. Sure, she valued fitness and truly believed what we espoused in the magazine, but I suspect she wasn't a big fan of gym class in junior high. She was active enough to stay healthy, and tried various classes at the health club to keep herself interested, but she'd never really been a jock. Exercise was a pleasant daily task, not much more.

We were also joined by another editor, Alexandra. Alexandra was quite athletic, a runner who occasionally ran in races. She came along to offer moral support for Ann and to learn how to walk fast enough to make it a workout. Then she'd be able to give her knees and ankles a break from the pounding of running by racewalking once in a while.

So guess what happened? We created a monster—but not the one you'd suspect. In the first session Ann and Alexandra learned the basics of racewalk technique, using my patented "kids scurrying at poolside" teaching method (hey, it works—but more on that later). They both did fine, but it seemed Ann had a natural knack for the movement. So at the end of the session I did a standard wrap-up drill: I spaced them out so that Alexandra had a bit of a lead for a short walking "sprint." I told Ann to try to catch her, then I dashed ahead to Alexandra and told her to just keep Ann at bay.

You'd have thought I'd used an electric cattle prod on Ann. She took off and chewed up the distance between them in no time. (Keep in mind that *Alexandra* was the experienced runner.) So I lined them up again, gave Alexandra a bigger lead, and had them take off. Again—*vroooom!*—Ann churned up next to Alexandra and blazed past. With a very determined look on her face, no less. A third sprint with an even larger lead for Alexandra only stoked Ann's competitive fires more—she cruised past driving her arms, breathing hard, and (I'm quite certain) suppressing a grin. Not because she was beating Alexandra—they're good friends (or at least, used to be)—but because she'd mastered the skill. She was succeeding. Dare I say, she was finding her inner athlete.

There are three pretty compelling lessons in this little story, which I've seen played out many times at my clinics around the country:

- **Walking really is for everyone.** Even very vigorous walking, fast enough to make it a challenging workout, is completely attainable whether you consider yourself an athlete or not.

- **Mastering the technique is key.** Even though Alexandra was very fit from running, it turns out that Ann's experiences in yoga and kickboxing classes may have helped her more, because she was accustomed to patiently working to master new skills. And developing good technique made her a faster walker sooner.

- **Everyone has an athlete inside.** You may be competitive and you may not, but everyone enjoys the thrill of mastering a physical challenge. As Roger Bannister suggests, we can all enjoy finding our own form of physical expression. Walking may be the best way to attain that simple joy; it's certainly the most accessible.

What the experts recommend

It's worth taking the time to find your athlete inside, because there's great value in adding fast walks to your routine. Way back in 1978 the American College of Sports Medicine (ACSM) released a position statement on how much exercise you need to truly be fit. The experts have updated it periodically over the years, but the recommendation basically has three points now:

1. Three to five days per week, exercise for 20 to 60 minutes at an intensity that sustains your heart rate at 60 to 90 percent of its maximum level. On days you exercise longer, err toward lower levels of intensity; during shorter workouts, work at higher levels of effort.
2. At least twice a week, do resistance training for all of your major muscle groups—for example, a routine of 8 to 10 exercises. Do 8 to 12 repetitions of each exercise, with a weight or resistance that's sufficient to cause fatigue by the last rep.
3. Most days of the week, include regular flexibility exercises (such as static stretching) to develop and maintain a healthy range of motion.

These are far more specific and demanding guidelines than the recommendation found in the surgeon general's 1996 report (at least 30 minutes of moderate physical activity most days of the week). I'm convinced that the difference has caused some of the confusion over recent years in the media and among the public at large. After all, it begs the question, "How much exercise do I really have to do?" That's what people really want to know. In fact, what most people are asking—some actually say it to me—is "How little exercise can I get away with?"

The real answer is: "It depends on what you want." That's because the two guidelines are directed at two very different goals. If you want to reduce your risk of disease, drop your cholesterol levels and blood pressure a bit, feel better when you wake up in the morning, and probably live longer and certainly better, the surgeon general's advice is enough for you: Shoot for at least 30 minutes per day. It's a recommendation targeted for improved *health*.

The Activity Pyramid

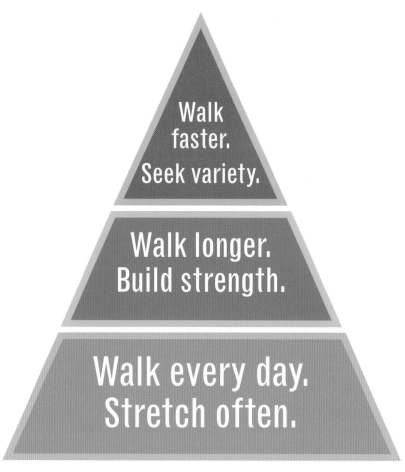

Walk
faster.
Seek variety.

Walk longer.
Build strength.

Walk every day.
Stretch often.

For total fitness, try for all the elements on the activity pyramid,
in proportion to their size.

However, if you want to really improve your *fitness,* then you need to tackle the more complete ACSM fitness guidelines. Meeting this higher standard will help you lose serious weight, build muscle tone and strength, change the shape of your body, and provide more noticeable improvements in your cardiovascular fitness. It will also require that you walk fast a couple of times a week. Only by challenging your muscular and cardiovascular systems will you make them that much stronger, and only by burning calories at a higher level can you make big changes in your body's shape. If you think back to the activity pyramid, you will recall that all of the above components are necessary to climb to the very top.

Why seek variety, too?

The top of the activity pyramid mentions the importance of seeking variety. This refers to occasionally searching out activities that help build your balance and coordination, too, because they're important components of total fitness. Balance is actually a skill that you can train and improve. Having good balance and coordination later in life, as well as muscular strength and

Walk Talk: Why should I be walking faster?

There are plenty of ways to boost your heart rate and burn more calories during a walk, but speeding up is the most straightforward and natural. You don't need any special equipment, facilities, or terrain; just master the basic elements of swift-walking techniques and you've got an intense workout anywhere you need it. Here are six reasons it's worth the effort at least two days a week:

1. Greater aerobic fitness. Whether you're dashing to catch a flight, sprinting after a six-year-old in backyard Capture the Flag, or striding through a weekend hike, you won't become winded when going all-out. You'll also be able to sustain a moderate level of effort for a longer time, since it'll feel so much easier.

2. You'll increase your speed. Only by getting near your body's speed limit can you begin to increase it. Occasional very fast walks will help make you a faster walker all the time.

3. You'll cover more ground. At 3 miles per hour, a 2-mile round trip to the convenience store takes 40 minutes; boost your speed to 4.5 miles per hour and you can make it in less than 25 minutes. Additional speed means greater range whether you're walking to work, for errands, or just for fun.

4. Greater strength. You'll develop power in your lower body that will help carry you up stairs and hills in the city, or scrambling over rocks and inclines on the trail.

5. More muscle and less fat. Walking at challenging speeds moves you into the serious calorie-burning range. You'll build more muscle tone and peel away the fat layers on top so that you (and others) can appreciate those muscles.

6. Improved health. Research at the Cooper Institute in Dallas, Texas, compared the health profiles and life spans of literally thousands of people whose fitness had been tested there over the years. What they found was in some ways astonishing—fitness was one of the best indicators of how long someone would live. You'd expect fitter people to live longer, but their research suggested that being fit is just as important as avoiding smoking and maintaining a healthy weight, two well-established factors in long-term health.

Good Balance and Coordination Builders

Vigorous Activities (at least 30 min. worth)	Moderate Activities (need 45 min. or more)	Recreational or Group Activities (need 60 min. or more)
High-intensity step class	Low-impact aerobics	Yoga, tai chi
In-line skating, fast	Volleyball (two-on-two, beach)	Volleyball (six-on-six, yard)
Vigorous dancing (ballet, modern)	Squash, racquetball	Ultimate Frisbee
One-on-one basketball	Tennis (singles)	Tennis (doubles)
Mountain biking (trails)	Road cycling (moderate)	Recreational bicycling
Kayaking (white water)	Kayaking (flat water)	Canoeing (recreational)
Jumping rope (20 min.)	Soccer (playing hard)	Golf (90 min.)

endurance, reduces your chance of falls or other accidental injuries. Improving your muscle coordination and control not only can make you a better athlete—whether in weekend softball or martial arts class—but will also make you less likely to slip on ice, pull a muscle lifting a child out of a car seat, or drop something on your head while putting groceries on the top shelf.

Do you need special exercises to work on your balance and coordination? Actually, you may already do things that help. For example, high-speed walking improves muscle coordination, and hiking on rough trails can challenge your balance. Lifting free weights or doing calisthenics also requires more balance and control than using a weight machine (which guides the weight for you).

On page 133 are some other activities that are good coordination builders—but they also can substitute for one of your walking workouts. The table shows how much you need to do for an activity to roughly equal a fast 30- to 40-minute walk. For more details on cross-training, see chapter 15.

You *can* have it all

To summarize your weekly goals:

- Two walks a week of 20 to 40 minutes at your fastest pace (usually better than 4.5 miles per hour).
- Three or four moderate walks of at least 45 to 60 minutes; make one even longer when you can (typically in the 3.5- to 4.5-mile-per-hour range)
- A moderate walk of 30 minutes on the remaining day (with one day off).
- Two or three days a week of strength training.
- A simple stretching routine at least five days a week.
- Occasional activities that challenge your balance and muscle coordination; they can replace a walk of similar length and intensity.

Don't panic! It still boils down to six or seven days of walking (or the equivalent) each week, two or three days of strength training, and fairly regular stretching.

Breathing hard is good for you

So why all this emphasis on faster walks? First, fast walks tax your body in ways that no amount of slow walking can. Second, you won't always have time for longer walks, so you should try to get as much as possible out of your shorter efforts. That happens if you go fast.

Your body basically utilizes energy in two ways. The most common way is aerobically, by using oxygen that you breathe into your lungs at a steady rate as you burn fuel. Known as aerobic metabolism, it's what you do when strolling at a comfortable, sustainable pace. But you also have a high-speed, high-energy system that works without oxygen, called anaerobic metabolism. Anaerobic metabolism kicks in when you do something that makes your muscles demand oxygen faster than you can breathe it in and get it to them. You use it more during short, demanding activities, and you can keep up this high-intensity energy production for only so long, depending on your fitness.

In daily life you use a mix of the two energy systems. Strolling easily at a pace that barely gets you breathing is almost entirely aerobic. Running fast up two flights of stairs, on the other hand, has a big anaerobic component. Here's the tricky part—in general you can build your high-intensity or anaerobic fitness only by stressing your body at high intensities. By "high" I mean doing things that get you breathing hard, but not necessarily buckled over with your hands on your knees ready to throw up.

Exercise scientists use complex measures like your heart rate, ventilation rate, and rate of oxygen consumption to determine how hard you're working when exercising. But they've also realized that people have a pretty good knack for recognizing their effort level just by how they feel—sort of the "hands on your knees ready to throw up" test. Researchers developed a scale, called the Rate of Perceived Exertion (RPE), that standardizes the sense of how hard you're working during exercise. That original scale is rated from 1 to 20, and word descriptions (such as "very light" and "extremely hard") are associated with the numeric values.

When talking about walking in a qualitative way, I've found that a simpler 1-to-10 scale works fine for most people. (Many physiologists now use this simpler scale.) It's shown opposite; I'll use it to help describe effort levels for various workouts. A 1 on the scale means your effort is very, very weak, essentially nonexistent. In other words, no more effort than sitting around watching television (and entirely aerobic production). As you move toward 10 the numbers represent higher levels of effort and, eventually, a greater proportion of anaerobic energy. A 3 might be barely walking at window-shopping pace; 5 is more like an

RPE	Description of Your Effort
0	Nothing at all
1	Very, very weak
2	Very weak
3	Moderate
4	Somewhat strong
5	Strong
6	Strong
7	Very strong
8	Very strong
9	Very strong
10	Very, very strong; maximal

The 1-to-10 scale for Rating of Perceived Exertion (RPE). This is a simple way to estimate how hard you're working that's consistent from one workout to the next.

easy, purposeful stroll, walking to get somewhere. An RPE of 7 is a hard enough effort that you couldn't sustain it for too long (say, 40 minutes), and 9 is downright pushing your speed limit. Working at 10, of course, is all-out—you barely feel you can take 10 more steps without having to stop.

Get in the habit of thinking about where you are on the RPE scale when you're out for a walk. It's a good tool to use in helping boost the intensity of your workouts a couple of times per week. Whenever possible—even if you're walking to work or the store for errands—your quick 20- to 40-minute walks (at the top of the pyramid) should rate 7 or more on the scale.

Check your fitness to start

Because you're now incorporating faster walks two or three days a week, it's worth taking stock of your fitness. But don't get stuck in the rut of thinking that your weight is the gold standard. Shedding some pounds may be your goal, and walking faster will certainly help get you there. But it's not going to tell you whether your heart is stronger or your legs can carry you longer and faster. For that, take this quick fitness quiz.

Quiz IV: At-Home Fitness Quiz

This simple quiz is a combination of subjective questions and more concrete assessments of your physical condition. The absolute value of your score is less important than seeing improvement over time. Take the test right now, then every 8 to 10 weeks to watch your fitness bloom.

Subjective Questions

1. If you had to carry two heavy (for you) bags of groceries up two flights of stairs, which best describes what you would do?
   a) Carry them both up and perhaps be breathing hard, but be fine.
   b) Carry them both up, but have to pause once, and really be tired on top.
   c) Try to carry them both, but have to stop and put one down for a break halfway up.
   d) Just carry one up at a time and still be very tired.
   e) Either find an elevator or have someone else do it.

2. Friends invite you to join them for a bike ride 5 miles to the next town to attend an outdoor concert you really want to see. Which best describes what you would do?
   a) Go and be able to pedal hard the whole way, shifting gears so you could pedal up and even *down* hills.
   b) Go and pedal most of the time, but coast all the downhills.
   c) Go and be able to pedal about half the time, but do a lot of coasting to rest.
   d) Go, but have to take it at a very leisurely pace, stopping for at least one break.
   e) Drive the car and meet them at the concert.

3. At an all-day picnic, family and friends are playing a rousing game of volleyball (or tennis, soccer, basketball—pick any fairly physical game you'd enjoy). Which best describes what you would do?
   a) Play all afternoon, pausing only to let someone else in or to eat or grab a drink now and then.
   b) Play for an hour or so, then call it a day.
   c) Play for 15 to 30 minutes here or there, but no more than an hour total.
   d) Jump in for one 20- to 30-minute spurt, at most.
   e) Just watch.

Score 5 points for an (a), 4 points for a (b), 3 for a (c), 2 for a (d), and 1 for an (e)

If you scored:

- **13 to 15.** Great. You can't improve much on your subjective score, so focus on performance improvements (the fitness tests below).
- **9 to 12.** Solid. Think about where your weaknesses are (strength? shorter hard efforts? sustained activities?) and focus on improving those in your exercise program.
- **6 to 8.** Fair. Try to hit the full range of exercise options to round out your fitness.
- **3 to 5.** Fear not—you have lots of room for improvement, but you'll see it if you stick with the program.

Fitness Tests

1. Check your resting heart rate.
   What it tests: Your baseline cardiovascular fitness.
   What to do: The first thing when you wake up in the morning—before you sit up or even roll over—take your pulse. Keep a clock with a second hand or a watch by the bed. Gently place your first two fingers on either side of your throat, moving them until you feel a distinct pulse. Count the number of pulses you feel in 10 seconds and multiply that number by 6. This will

give you the number of beats your heart takes per minute (BPM). Check it three days in a row, and average the results.

What it means: A low resting heart rate indicates greater cardiac strength and overall fitness. Typical numbers:

Less than 50 beats a minute	**Like a real athlete**
50 to 60 beats a minute	**Very fit**
60 to 75 beats a minute	**Average**
More than 75 beats a minute	**Room for improvement**

If your number is high, consider more longer walks to continue building endurance and overall aerobic conditioning. However, you can expect your resting heart rate to change only about five beats per minute or so overall; much of resting heart rate is genetically predetermined.

2. Walk a 1-mile time trial.

What it tests: Aerobic/anaerobic fitness and endurance.

What to do: Head to a local high school or college track, do the warm-up moves from the end of chapter 1 (see page 6), then walk easily for 15 minutes. Once you're warmed up, walk four laps as fast as you can, trying to sustain an even pace (not sprinting at the end). Record your exact time for 1 mile.

What it means: If you push yourself hard, this is a great test of both your endurance and your high-intensity (anaerobic) energy systems. Typical times:

Less than 11 minutes	**Give the U.S. national team a call**
11 to 14 minutes	**Very fit**
14 to 19 minutes	**Average**
More than 19 minutes	**Room for improvement**

Bursts of fast walking, for as little as 2 minutes up to as much as 30, will improve this score.

3. Stand up/sit down test.

What it tests: Muscular strength, balance, and coordination.

What to do: Place a straight-backed chair without a cushion against a wall. Begin this test sitting upright with your feet flat on the floor, your back touching the back of the chair, and your arms folded across your chest, hands on opposite shoulders. Then count how many times you can rise to a full standing position and return to your seat in exactly 20 seconds. Keep your arms folded, make sure your back touches the chair back every time, and go as fast as you can. (Warm up before doing this test—it's fairly demanding if you really go hard.)

What it means: This short but sweet test challenges your strength, coordination, and pure anaerobic power—you barely have time to get breathing hard before it's over. Typical numbers:

More than 20	**Super-jock (are you sure you did them right?)**
13 to 19	**Very fit**
6 to 12	**Average**
5 or fewer	**Room for improvement**

This requires skill as well as fitness—the total-body strength routine and some upper- and lower-body cross-training activities (see chapter 15 for both) will improve this score.

13

Technique for Building Speed

Breaking a sweat, breathing hard, and boosting your heart rate are all great—in theory. But walking fast enough to make your heart pound isn't necessarily easy. People have even told me that it's just not possible to walk fast enough to really get the heart pumping. You know you could run fast enough to soak a shirt with sweat, but walking much beyond a slight "glow" might seem out of the question. It's not the activity that's preventing you from working harder, it's your technique. How do I know? Because competitive racewalkers sustain speeds well over 8 miles an hour for either 12-mile (men and women) or 31-mile (men) races—walking, and physiological testing shows them to be among the fittest people on the planet. By stealing a few simple tips from them, you can certainly handle 4.5 miles per hour.

Once you relax, fast-walking technique should come fairly naturally. Hopefully you've already tried working on improving your posture and taking faster steps. The additional core elements of fast walking—bending your arms and pushing off your toes—are what humans do naturally when forced to walk faster with no formal instruction. This has been shown in the laboratory with people walking on treadmills, but a better "experiment" is one we've all seen.

Think of the last time you were at a swimming pool with lots of young children. Invariably they start running around the deck—probably chasing the kid who grabbed the inflatable two-headed horse. The lifeguard's whistle squeals, and he shouts, "Hey you kids, no running. *Walk* on the pool deck!" So they all break into a walk—as fast a walk as they can muster. (After all, they *need* that two-headed horse.) Think about what their walk looks like: very upright posture, extremely quick steps, bent arms swinging vigorously front to back. But nobody said to them, "Okay you kids, here's how to walk super-fast so you can catch Homer when he takes the horse." Someone said, "Walk," they wanted to go fast, and this is what they did. So don't doubt you can do it—just don't think *too* hard, and let it happen.

It still starts with posture

Faster walking starts with sound posture—just as in most other sports. Whether you're swinging a golf club or tennis racket, shooting a free throw, paddling a canoe, or simply trying to bust a 13-minute mile (about 4.6 miles per hour), having your body aligned in the right position can make all the difference. So even though I urged you to master a "tall" posture at moderate walking speeds, it should still be your first concern when walking fast. Then add the other elements below.

Walk as tall as you can

Maintain an upright but comfortable posture and you'll keep your rib cage open for easier breathing; your lower back and hips will also be well positioned for a quick, powerful stride. A slouch or roll in your shoulders, a forward lean from the hips, or an arch in your lower back can all undermine these elements of walking power.

Tips:

- Have your head level, and gaze forward. Drop only your eyes to check your footing; don't lower your chin.
- Relax your neck, back, and shoulders.
- Keep your stomach muscles gently contracted and your back fairly flat.

As fast as your feet can go

The absolute critical variable for fast walking is faster steps. On your fastest walks consider counting steps occasionally, with a goal of at least 135 steps a minute. When you've mastered that, set 150 steps per minute as your next goal.

Tips:

- Make comfortable strides so your feet touch down practically beneath you, not out in front.
- Focus on smooth, quick steps, and think about pulling your leg forward as quickly as you can as soon as your foot leaves the ground.

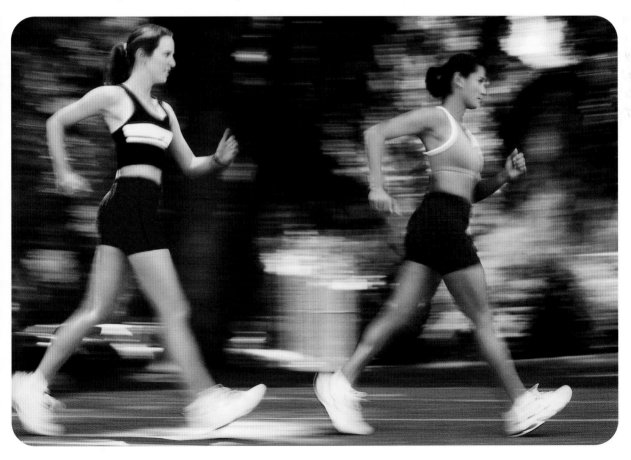

Fast arms make fast feet

The best way to ensure that you maintain quick strides is a very powerful, compact, and quick arm swing. The arms and legs will always move in synchrony, and faster arms will make faster legs.

A key to getting the fastest possible arm swing is bending your arms 90 degrees. That makes your arm a shorter pendulum, and a shorter pendulum swings faster than a long one. For a reminder, think of the weight that hangs down on the pendulum of a grandfather clock. The height is adjustable to control the accuracy of the clock. The man at my local clock repair shop told me the simple rule they remember: "Lower is slower." Lower the weight and make the pendulum longer, and it swings more slowly—exactly what you *don't* want to happen when you're trying to walk faster. So you should bend your arms when walking and running fast to shorten the pendulum, and help them swing faster.

Tips:

- Bend your arms as much as—but no more than—a right angle.
- Keep the elbow fixed (imagine it's in a cast); don't let your elbow swing open and closed as the arm swings.
- Have your hands trace an arc from waistband height (on the backswing) to chest height (in front).
- Allow your hands to come to the centerline of your body, but not to cross it in front.

Walk Talk: Sometimes I feel some tightness or soreness in my lower back, especially when walking faster. What can I do?

Back pain should never be treated lightly, because it can be severely debilitating if it becomes a chronic problem. If back pain persists, be sure to see a doctor. In general, many experts now agree that maintaining muscular fitness and moderate activity levels are crucial parts of treatment for back pain.

The naturally longer stride and greater muscular demands of faster walking can certainly trigger lower-back tightness, especially if your abdominal muscles aren't very fit. That's why it's important to regularly do the full torso-strengthening routine shown in chapter 4 (or the full strength routine in chapter 15). But you should also be thinking about gently contracting your abdominal muscles while walking. Nothing severe—just the feeling of firming and tucking your belly in a bit.

Do the Posture Check

This move will help you get accustomed to the feeling of firming your stomach muscles, so you can do this naturally while walking. Stand with the back of your head, shoulders, and feet against a wall. Slide one hand behind the small of your back, in the natural arch you'll find there. Now gently contract your abdominal muscles—just firming and tucking your belly muscles—and feel your back flatten against your hand. You don't have to get your back entirely flat against the wall—a certain amount of arch in the back is very normal. But work hard enough to feel your back push against your hand if you can.

Make the Posture Check an Exercise

To build some abdominal fitness and control, repeat this move several times before or after your walk. Tighten the stomach muscles, feel the back flatten somewhat, and hold for 10 seconds. Then relax for 5 seconds. Repeat 2 more times. Work up to being able to tighten for 6 holds of 10 seconds each. Then try to string them into longer holds (4 of 15 seconds, 3 of 20 seconds), eventually tightening for a minute straight.

Pushing off for power

Generating a lot of push at the end of each step helps in two ways—you produce more forward drive with each stride, and you help prepare your leg to swing forward quickly as soon as it leaves the ground. And that's important to maintaining a very quick stride. The very tip of your toe should be the last thing to leave the ground on each step. Here's a sign that you're doing it right: You should be able to see wear on the bottom of your shoe all the way up to your big toe. If not, you're not pushing off enough.

Tips:

- Feel your foot roll smoothly from the heel all the way through the toes.
- Consciously push off with your toes at the end of every step.
- Feel like you're showing someone behind you the sole of your shoe at the end of each step.

Use these techniques to boost your speed anytime you're walking—not just during hard workouts. Other than bending your arms, these all work for a quick stroll to the corner store or even walking from the parking lot to the office.

Improving technique on the treadmill

Though it's important to always be aware of healthy walking technique, sometimes it's easiest to make improvements by focusing only on your walking. The treadmill is a great place to do that—it's a smooth surface, you're moving at an even tempo, and you can really just pay attention to what you're doing. Here are three workouts to help put all these technique tips into practice.

1. The tech check.

The goal: Efficient walking technique.

The workout: Walk at paces from easy to taxing with mirrors to the front and sides to check your technique (or set the 'mill at a 45-degree angle to the mirrored wall, to glimpse your side view without craning your neck). Look for tall, relaxed posture, elbows bent no more than 90 degrees, and an aggressive push off your toes. Want to get really high-tech? Set a video camera on yourself, and display it on a television right in front of you. Then make adjustments while you walk.

2. The quick step.

The goal: Improved foot speed (and reduced boredom).

The workout: After an ample warm-up, count your steps for one minute, then walk moderately for two. Crank up the machine until you hit 140 strides per minute on the pickups, 115 on the recoveries; keep adding 5 to each as your skill and fitness improve. Repeat at least 5 times (or just 2 or 3 if you do this at the end of another workout).

3. The retro

The goal: Coordination, balance, and strength.

The workout: Simply walk backward on the treadmill at an easy pace for two to five minutes at a time. Intersperse this during or at the end of another workout; it reverses the firing of your muscles and gives your neural system a change, too. When you go back to normal walking, you'll feel stronger and *very* coordinated.

If you feel you have to try a treadmill—say, because you really want to work on technique—
but you can't seem to get motivated, consider one of these tips:

1. **Walk with a friend.** Choose a quick-but-conversational pace on side-by-side treadmills at the health club or Y (or in your basement, if you decide to invest together).
2. **Walk meditatively.** Light candles (or even incense), put on your most calming music, focus on the rhythm of your steps, and walk your stress away at a comfortable pace.
3. **Make it a tale of the tape.** Set a small recorder nearby. With no distractions and plenty of blood flowing to your brain, you can dictate memos, grocery lists, research papers, or the Great American Novel while you walk. Or reverse the process: Master another language by listening to language CDs.
4. **Create a breeze.** Set up a fan in front of the treadmill, to get some of the sense and cooling of walking outdoors.
5. **Circle the globe.** Log your mileage each day or week on a map mounted by your treadmill. Walk across your state, across the country, or even around the world.

Five common technique errors and how to fix them

How hard can it really be? It's only walking, after all. Left foot, right foot, left . . . right? After millions of years of evolutionary training, we should be pretty good at our preferred gait. Yet some folks look downright silly when they try to elevate their walking to a calorie-burning speed. What makes such a familiar activity so hard when you try to turn it into a workout?

First, blame bad postural habits and movement patterns. They're caused by everything from slouching at a computer keyboard or while reading (you just straightened up, didn't you?) to carting a child on one hip or a golf bag over one shoulder. They wreak havoc with your posture over time. Second, there's the "trying-too-hard" syndrome. In trying to walk faster, people make their walk into a caricature. They adopt exaggerated arm swings, extra-long strides, and energetic hip gyrations all in the name of speed.

Unfortunately, such techniques aren't just aesthetically aggravating; they also limit your speed and your workout. Worse, they can lead to discomfort and injury if your gaffe is grand enough. So give your own technique the once-over. Whether you watch yourself in a storefront window or hop on a treadmill in front of a mirror, watch out for these five common errors, and apply the corrections as needed.

Error 1. Looking for spare change. Head down, shoulders slouched.

Likely candidates: Anyone who lives at the keyboard or behind a steering wheel.

Warning signs: Tightness and fatigue in the upper back, neck, and shoulders.

How to fix it?

- Get your eyes on the horizon. If your gaze is off in the distance, not down at your own feet or the ground just in front of you, that will tend to pull your whole body more upright.

- Pull your shoulders back and chest forward. (The marines are right.)

Error 2. Goose-stepping. Taking an extra-long stride.

Likely candidates: The followers of instructors who urge you "reach for your stride."

Warning signs: Sore shins, tightness in the hamstrings (back of the thigh), and a jarring thud on every step.

How to fix it?

- Think rolling, not bouncing, from one stride to the next. Try to put your foot down as fast as you can.
- Don't reach for the longest possible stride, and don't let your heels slam into the ground on each step.
- Feel your body glide along the ground, not bounce up and down. If someone saw only your head over a hedge, it should look like you're riding a bike, not running.

Error 3. Chicken wings. Elbows flailing out to the sides with each arm swing.

Likely candidates: Speed aspirants, especially those trying to figure out racewalking.

Warning signs: You can't walk near a wall or a partner without banging an elbow.

How to fix it?

- Feel your thumb rub the waistband of your pants as your hand swings back, then stop it there. (Don't let it swing any farther back).
- Imagine you're trying to elbow someone directly behind you.
- Don't let your hips have an exaggerated side-to-side sashay.
- Walk very near a wall or hedge—the closer, the better. Negative reinforcement will help you tuck your elbows in.

Error 4. Shelf-butt. Excessive arch in the lower back, causing your rear end to lag behind.

Likely candidates: Those with weak stomach muscles.

Warning signs: Tightness in the lower back and upper gluteal muscles.

How to fix it? Do the "posture check" (see the box on page 140: stand against a wall and flatten your belly) before heading out for your walk.

- Keep your rear end tucked underneath you; consciously pull it under you by gently tightening your stomach muscles and flattening your belly.

Error 5. Boxing. Driving the arms high—to shoulder height or above—in front.

Likely candidates: Everyone trying to improve their upper-body workout or drive their arms for greater speed.

Warning signs: A choppy stride and seeing your hands swing up into view on every step.

How to fix it?

- Think about a quick, compact arm swing.
- In front, your hands should come up only to chest height—if you're looking forward, that's just into your peripheral vision but no higher.
- Don't open and close the angle of your elbow on each arm swing; imagine the elbow is fixed in a cast at a 90-degree angle.

Because she's so fit and full of energy, you'd have no problem believing that Laney Hixon, a nutritionist and weight-loss counselor, had been a high school cheerleader. What you might not accept so readily is that after her first year of college she put on at least 30 pounds. The complex reasons were not something to cheer about: more schoolwork, less physical activity (she used to walk regularly), hit-and-miss eating habits, and issues of self-esteem.

The Turning Point

"It was coming home from college for a high school football game weighing, well, I-won't-tell-you-how-much, and realizing that my friends and family were surprised how I looked," says Laney. Her homecoming shocked her into deciding that she was going to straighten out her disordered eating and start walking again. In doing so, she began to study nutrition and in time became a registered dietitian. At the same time she kicked up her walking a few notches, making it more and more athletic. After settling in Atlanta for work, she hooked up with a local racewalking instructor (Bonnie Stein, now in Boca Raton, Florida) and *really* ramped up her walking up to the next level.

A Week in Her Life

Although Laney claims not to be a serious racewalker, it's clear she uses elements of the technique to make many of her walks serious workouts. Because she's kept so busy at the hospital where she works, some of her workouts have to be fairly short. To compensate, she uses speed to make sure those are serious calorie burners. On the weekends she does have time for at least one longer, hour-plus walk.

Her Biggest Accomplishment

By sharing her personal experience with others, Laney can help them realize that walking provides more than physical benefits—it also has emotional benefits capable of turning their lives around. "Many of the folks who come to me have self-image issues. They've been made fun of and feel horrible about themselves. They have to deal with that before we even start on serious diet and exercise." But starting to walk—even 5 and 10 minutes a day—gives many that first sense of beginning to take control.

Her Key to Success

Laney practices what she preaches, having been there.

	Date	Today's Activity Goal(s)	Total Minutes (or √)	Stretch? (√)	Comments, Other Activities? (vigorous chores, sports, other exercise, etc.)	Estimated Miles Walked
Sunday		30				
Monday		50, upper/lower				
Tuesday		45				
Wednesday		1:00				
Thursday		45, upper/lower				
Friday		off				
Saturday		1:15				

Miles this week: _____

Total miles for the year: _____

Mix up the intensity

Now that you'll begin adding even speedier walks to your week, you should try to make sure you vary your faster and slower days. But keep it simple: Just record how each day felt (*E* for easy, *M* for medium, *H* for hard), and try not to have more than two hard days in a row. Also, begin combining the upper- and lower-body strength routines into just two strength workouts a week if you haven't done so already. (They're shown on Monday and Thursday.) This is in preparation for moving to the next strength program in a few weeks.

Tip for the week. **Pick out a walking event to try in week 40. Check out the plethora of contacts under "Events" in the resource list at the end of this book, but also ask walking friends if they know of any fun, well-organized 5K walks coming up. (Of course, it's fine if you choose an event on a weekend near, but not exactly in, week 40.)**

	Date	Today's Activity Goal(s)	Total Minutes (or √)	Stretch? (√)	Comments, Other Activities? (vigorous chores, sports, other exercise, etc.)	Estimated Miles Walked
Sunday		cross-train				
Monday		50, upper/lower				
Tuesday		40				
Wednesday		1:00				
Thursday		45, upper/lower				
Friday		off				
Saturday		1:30				

Miles this week: _____

Total miles for the year: _____

Consciously add cross-training to your week

This section of the program promises to bring you all the components of fitness: endurance, speed, strength, flexibility, balance, and coordination. To really attain all of these, you need to add one more element to your routine of long and fast walks, stretching, and strengthening. On alternate Sundays I'll begin recommending cross-training. Read (or reread) chapter 15 for background on the importance of doing other activities—anything from tennis to tango classes—to build balance, coordination, and well-rounded fitness.

Tip for the week. **Shoot for 30 to 60 minutes of cross-training on the days it's recommended. Be sure to begin unfamiliar activities gradually, to reduce the risk of injury. In fact, it's often best—the most fun and least frustrating—to attend some demonstrations or take a class before trying an entirely new sport or activity.**

	Date	Today's Activity Goal(s)	Total Minutes (or √)	Stretch? (√)	Comments, Other Activities? (vigorous chores, sports, other exercise, etc.)	Estimated Miles Walked
Sunday		40				
Monday		45, upper/lower				
Tuesday		50				
Wednesday		1:00, 1-mile test				
Thursday		45, upper/lower				
Friday		off				
Saturday		1:00				

Miles this week: _____

Total miles for the year: _____

See how fast you can walk a mile

On Wednesday (or whichever day works best with your schedule) plan to take your walk at a track. The goal is to determine your fastest time for walking a mile—a good indicator of your overall fitness and walking strength. Record your time here in the exercise log. Over the next several weeks, the program is going to incorporate workouts designed to improve your walking speed, to help you prepare for walking in a short event (5K or so) in week 40, and longer one (10K or more) in week 48. As part of your preparations, you'll check your 1-mile walking time again in eight weeks to see how you're improving.

Tip for the week. **Walk easily for 15 minutes to warm up, then walk 1 mile (four laps of the track) as fast as you can. Try to maintain the fastest pace you can for the entire mile—don't start slowly and sprint at the finish. Notice your time for the mile, then walk easily in the outer lanes of the track to cool down, for a total walking time of one hour. For a real boost, ask a friend to time you—it should help motivate you to your best time.**

	Date	Today's Activity Goal(s)	Total Minutes (or √)	Stretch? (√)	Comments, Other Activities? (vigorous chores, sports, other exercise, etc.)	Estimated Miles Walked
Sunday		cross-train				
Monday		45, upper/lower				
Tuesday		35				
Wednesday		1:00, speed #1				
Thursday		30, upper/lower				
Friday		off				
Saturday		2:00 hike				

Miles this week: _____

Total miles for the year: _____

Build speed with Wednesday workouts and strength with Saturday hikes

Of course, you don't have to do them on Wednesday, but it's time to sprinkle the speed workouts described in chapter 14 into your weeks. There are eight workouts (numbered 1 to 8), and I'll recommend you try another one each week. So if you haven't read chapter 14 yet, or if it's been a while, take a look at those workouts.

You'll also see occasional hikes of two hours or more showing up on the weekends. These are great strength builders, and they give your body and mind a break. Pull out your hiking gear (now that you're a seasoned pro) and enjoy some relaxing time on the trail.

Tip for the week. Speed workout #1, the "out and back" workout, is scheduled on Wednesday this week. Hook up with some walking friends if you can, but even if you have to do it alone make it a hard effort. Walk an out-and-back course, heading out at a fast pace. After 20 minutes turn around and retrace your steps, trying to go faster than you did going out!

Date	Today's Activity Goal(s)	Total Minutes (or √)	Stretch? (√)	Comments, Other Activities? (vigorous chores, sports, other exercise, etc.)	Estimated Miles Walked
Sunday	40				
Monday	50, strength				
Tuesday	45				
Wednesday	1:00, speed #2				
Thursday	30, strength				
Friday	off				
Saturday	1:15				

Miles this week: ——————

Total miles for the year: ——————

Start the new strength-training routine

In chapter 15 a more advanced version of the strength-training routine is introduced. Now's the time to take your healthier, stronger body to the next level with more total-body exercises that will enhance your coordination as well as your strength. Don't hesitate to get help or instruction (say, at a gym or with a couple of visits with a personal trainer) if you're not comfortable with any of the moves.

Tip for the week. **On days when you're pressed for time and can't get in both a walk and strength training as scheduled, try this trick: circuit training. Create a "circuit" of the exercises in your routine, and move quickly from one to the next. Do one exercise for 30 seconds, then rest for 30 seconds as you get ready for the next move. With increasing fitness you can go to 40 seconds on, 20 seconds off; move through the full routine twice. I guarantee that you'll find it a challenging and efficient aerobic and strength workout.**

	Date	Today's Activity Goal(s)	Total Minutes (or √)	Stretch? (√)	Comments, Other Activities? (vigorous chores, sports, other exercise, etc.)	Estimated Miles Walked
Sunday		cross-train				
Monday		50, strength				
Tuesday		45				
Wednesday		1:00, speed #3				
Thursday		40, strength				
Friday		off				
Saturday		1:30				

Miles this week: _____

Total miles for the year: _____

Speed workouts really *will* speed you up

As well as the designated speed workouts on Wednesday, you should consciously make Monday a fast-walking day, too. The format is simple—begin with 10 minutes of easy walking to warm up, and plan for an easy 10 minutes to cool down. Everything in between—set your shoes on fire! Well, at least work at a fast enough pace that you really feel like you've worked hard when you're done. You're not buckled over gasping, but you're happy that you're finished.

Tip for the week. Remember the keys to faster walking: tall posture, faster steps, bent arms, and pushing off the toes. Try counting steps near the beginning, middle, and end of the fast part of your Monday walk to see if you're maintaining your speed. Count your steps for just 20 seconds (and multiply by 3 if you want steps per minute)—your goal should be to keep your step rate high throughout the speedy part of the walk.

	Date	Today's Activity Goal(s)	Total Minutes (or √)	Stretch? (√)	Comments, Other Activities? (vigorous chores, sports, other exercise, etc.)	Estimated Miles Walked
Sunday		40				
Monday		30, strength				
Tuesday		40				
Wednesday		1:00, speed #4				
Thursday		30				
Friday		off				
Saturday		2:30 hike				

Miles this week: ⎯⎯⎯⎯⎯⎯

Total miles for the year: ⎯⎯⎯⎯⎯⎯

Mix strength training into your speed workouts

Speed workout #4 is recommended for Wednesday. It's a version of circuit training (described in week 37) that combines brisk walking and strength exercises. You'll alternate 2 minutes of brisk walking with 30 seconds of a strength move for 15 minutes at a time. As a result, you don't have a second strength workout scheduled during the week—just on Monday, and as part of your speed workout on Wednesday. (So don't say I never did anything for you!)

Tip for the week. **Don't try to push the speed on your trail hikes. Because you're subjecting your body to plenty of high-intensity effort during the Monday and Wednesday speed workouts, you don't need to pound yourself on your hike. The mere fact that you're walking on rough terrain boosts the intensity of your workout anyway, and you really should let it be a completely relaxing outing.**

Date	Today's Activity Goal(s)	Total Minutes (or √)	Stretch? (√)	Comments, Other Activities? (vigorous chores, sports, other exercise, etc.)	Estimated Miles Walked
Sunday	cross-train				
Monday	55, strength				
Tuesday	35				
Wednesday	1:00, speed #5				
Thursday	40, strength				
Friday	off				
Saturday	1:05, speed #8				

Miles this week: _____

Total miles for the year: _____

Blaze through a 5K walk

Speed workout #8 is scheduled for this weekend. Hopefully you've signed up for the event ahead of time—take a look at some of the event-day tips in chapter 16 (see page 194) if you're not sure about the details. The most important thing, of course, is to have a good time.

Tip for the week. Try to hook up with someone experienced in walking in events if this is your first effort. Also, be sure to start at a reasonable pace—don't try walking faster than you've ever walked before.

Walking Speed (mph)	Minutes to Walk 1 Mile (min:sec)	Approximate Time for 5K (min:sec)
3.0	20:00	62:10
3.5	17:10	53:15
4.0	15:00	46:35
4.5	13:20	41:25
5.0	12:00	37:15
5.5	10:55	33:55
6.0	10:00	31:05

14

Workouts to Build Your Speed

Making haste patiently

If you're used to walking at a brisk but comfortable pace (say, from 3.5 to 4 miles per hour, or 18 to 15 minutes per mile), then don't expect to head out tomorrow, apply your new lessons in technique, and suddenly light the sidewalk on fire. Good technique is the key to going faster, but you're going have to build the fitness to maintain that technique. That leads to a chicken-and-egg question. You want to walk faster because it helps build fitness and strength. But you have to be more fit and stronger to maintain a faster walking pace. So which comes first: faster walks, or the fitness to sustain them?

They come together, of course, a little bit at a time. You have to do two things simultaneously—improve your walking technique and start to tackle faster speeds for short, but progressively longer, chunks of your walks.

Walking efficiently

You can improve the efficiency and power of your walking technique in two ways. First, get in the habit of thinking about better walking technique all the time. Even on your slowest, most relaxing walks or while warming up at a comfortable pace, remember to maintain good, tall posture and a quick, efficient stride. Try to make the cues (eyes on the horizon, quick steps, smooth roll from heel to toe) so familiar that you think of them whenever you're walking.

Second, begin to focus on specific elements of improved technique during your faster walks. Start by doing it one element at a time—thinking first about looking forward, not down. Then focus on quicker steps. This keeps it from becoming overwhelming, and helps you recognize which cues work for you. Over time, you can begin to put them all together on your fast walks.

Intervals: faster in little bits

Once you've begun gradually improving your technique at familiar speeds, it's time for a new adventure: speed work. There are all sorts of names and ways that speed is incorporated into walking (and running) workouts: intervals, tempo work, time trials, fartlek. That last word is Swedish for "speed play," and you'll know you're getting hardcore when you say it and don't understand why people giggle. ("Yeah, honey, I'm pretty tired; I lifted weights this morning and then did my 3-mile loop with some fartlek. Hey, what are you laughing at?")

The basic idea is to incorporate segments of faster walking into your workout, with walking at a comfortable speed before, after, and in between the speedy stuff. The fast segments have to be short enough that you can really boost your speed, but long enough that you get some conditioning effect—for your fitness to improve, your heart rate has to climb somewhat during your speedy segments. For a single week, a good approach is to mix in fairly short but very speedy segments on one day, and work on a more sustained but less speedy effort on another.

Got an hour?
Get in shape

Here are eight ideas guaranteed to optimize your training time and boost your walking speed. Designed for active walkers—and not the fainthearted—they all total an hour, and they'll make 60 minutes fly by faster than you can say, "Mike Wallace and Morley Safer." They're listed roughly from the least intense to the most. The early ones fit into your moderate 45- to 60-minute slots in the weekly plan; the later workouts are great for your pure speed walks.

Each workout is shown with running time, from 00 to 60 minutes, telling you exactly when to begin and end each segment. Of course, if you've got more or less time you can modify them accordingly—just use the frameworks laid out here.

#1. Out and back.

How: On a familiar out-and-back course with one or more walking pals of any ability; use the clock to guide how far you go and to balance your abilities.

Why: A great sustained workout that lets walkers of very different speeds challenge one another by turning around at a certain *time,* not distance.

00 to 10	Walk easily together to warm up.
10 to 30	Start your watches together, and head out on your predetermined course (make sure everyone knows it) at a pace you feel you can just barely sustain for 35 minutes. Don't worry about your partners if you spread out; walk at your own hard pace (a 6 to 7 RPE).
30 to 50	After exactly 20 minutes outbound, everyone turns around wherever they are and starts blazing back toward the starting point. Abilities are now equalized; the slower walkers outbound now have a head start for the return trip. The race is on!
50 to 55	Easy cool-down stroll.
55 to 60	Stretch.

#2. Hike it up.

How: Head up a long, moderate to steep uphill trail—a hiking trail or snow-free ski slope is ideal.

Why: Builds some of the leg strength and aerobic power needed for faster walking, even before you can go fast.

00 to 10	Start uphill easily to warm up, gradually increasing your pace.
10 to 30	Speed up to your hardest sustainable pace (about 7 RPE); pump your arms for added lift. (Lack a large hill? Then do continuous hard-up/easy-down laps on the longest incline you can find, or duplicate the continuous uphill effort on a treadmill with a 5 to 15 percent grade.)
30 to 55	Head back downhill, walking easily to cool down.
55 to 60	Stretch (especially thighs and buttocks).

#3. Climb the ladder.

How: Head to the track for a series of alternating fast and slow intervals that increase in length as you "climb the ladder."

Why: Long speedy intervals are critical to teaching your body to sustain faster speeds.

00 to 50	Start with two easy laps to warm up. Then do one lap fast (an RPE of about 8), one lap easy (4 or 5 RPE); two laps fast, two easy; and three laps fast, three easy. The total is 3.5 miles. This should leave you with 5 to 10 minutes for stretching. But if you're so speedy that it's not enough to fill an hour, bump up just the hard efforts by a lap: two fast, one easy; three fast, two easy; and four fast, three easy.
50 to 60	Stretch.

#4. Muscle and wind.

How: Walk along a par course trail with exercise stations or at a track with bleachers or benches available, and intersperse strength exercises between intervals of fast walking.

Why: A combination aerobic and strength workout that boosts both lung and muscle power.

00 to 10	Walk easily to warm up.
10 to 25	Pick up to a fast pace—enough to boost your breathing noticeably (at least a 7 RPE). After two minutes of walking, stop and work at one of the exercise stations for 30 seconds. (Don't worry about how many repetitions you do; just try to be working for most of the 30 seconds.) Then resume fast walking, stopping every two minutes for an exercise. Do this cycle six times. (Without exercise stations, just do these exercises: push-ups, abdominal crunches, isometric side supports, lunges, dips, and modified planks. See chapter 15.)
25 to 30	Walk easily to recover. No exercises; just catch your breath.
30 to 45	Repeat the two-minute fast walk/30-second exercise cycle 6 more times.
45 to 55	Walk easily to cool down.
55 to 60	Stretch.

#5. Who's in first?

How: A playful workout on any course with at least three walking buddies (but the more, the better—it's ideal for a club or team workout). You walk single file and take turns sprinting to the lead.

Why: A workout with short bursts of speed for improved anaerobic strength that uses your partners for motivation.

00 to 10	Group warm-up stroll, progressing gently to a brisk pace.
10 to 25	String out into single file, at least 20 yards from first to last. Walk at a brisk, no-nonsense, but not gut-busting pace (RPE of 7). Then the last walker in line pours on the speed until she passes first place (RPE of 9-plus for the sprint). As soon as she settles back into the pace at the head of the line, the new last-placer takes off for the front; keep cycling through.
30 to 35	Walk easily as a group for a break.
35 to 45	String out again, with the last walker again bursting to the front. But now each time a new walker takes the lead, try to continue at an ever-so-slightly faster pace. Over time, the whole group should pick up the tempo and be plenty ready to stop after 10 minutes.
45 to 55	Easy cool-down walk.
55 to 60	Stretch.

#6. Burn the straights.

How: Walk at a track with bursts of high speed on the straightaways.

Why: A challenging speed builder that lets you really focus on your best technique.

00 to 15	Walk easily to warm up in the outer lanes.
15 to 35	Keep circling the track, walking your fastest on the straightaways (a 9 RPE), cruising comfortably on the turns (no stopping). Focus on good technique and super-quick steps on the straights, even if your legs start to feel heavy.
35 to 45	Reverse direction and walk easily to cool down.
45 to 55	Two sets each of 10 push-ups, 20 abdominal crunches, and 10 dips. (Can't do all the calisthenics? Break them into smaller sets and do as many as you can!)
55 to 60	Stretch.

#7. Spring into action.

How: Sprinkle some jogging and running into your workout on a grassy athletic field or park (to reduce the impact).

Why: For an intense aerobic workout and putting some spring and power into your legs.

00 to 15	Warm-up walk, accelerating gradually to a brisk pace.
15 to 25	Cover 12 lengths of a football field (100 yards), repeating the following cycle 4 times: Walk 100 yards comfortably; cover the next 100 yards at a medium jog; then crank up to a run at full stride for the final 100 yards.
25 to 30	Five minutes of easy walking.
30 to 40	Repeat the walk-jog-run cycle 4 more times.
40 to 50	Easy cool-down walk.
50 to 60	Stretch.

#8. Crush the competition.

How: Jump into a 3-mile or 5K (3.1-mile) road race for a quality workout.

Why: Nothing makes you work like some healthy competition. If you're into serious workouts, there's a good chance you can walk 3 miles in less than an hour. The question is, how much less? Walk a 5K road race to find out—I guarantee you won't be the only walker there.

00 to 10	Easy stroll to loosen up.
10 to 55(?)	Walk the race at your fastest sustainable pace. Set a goal of beating at least a few runners.
55 to 60	Stroll easily and stretch. If your race runs more than an hour, don't skip stretching. Just walk faster next time! For more detailed information on road racing, see chapter 16.

Your heart doesn't lie

Timing yourself or estimating your speed with your step rate (chapter 8) and thinking about your Rate of Perceived Exertion are perfectly reasonable ways to try to make sure you're boosting your workout well into the fitness-building range. But they'll never be as accurate as simply measuring your heart rate. It's the gold standard, because it truly represents your physiological effort level, with no estimation error (counting steps to get speed, for example) or subjective element (as with RPE).

Most exercise recommendations are based on elevating your exercise heart rate to a certain percentage of your maximum heart rate; for example, 65 to 75 percent of maximum heart rate for moderate weight-loss walks. This means that to use it effectively, you have to know or be able to accurately estimate your maximum heart rate. There are a variety of formulas available for estimating maximum heart rate, and the more accuracy you want, the more complicated the formula. Here's a simple one that's widely used; it takes into account the fact that your maximum heart rate tends to drop as you get older.

Women: 226 - your age = maximum heart rate   (in beats per minute)
Men: 220 - your age = maximum heart rate

Walk Talk: Do I need a special watch for timing my workouts, especially now that I'm trying to go faster?

There is an almost overwhelming array of sport and outdoor watches available for people into active living. So how do you pick one? Don't get sucked in by extra features or fancy prices. Instead, think about the features you'll actually use and a look you'll be comfortable wearing.

Your first choice is between an analog watch—you know, like Mickey, with hands that go around a face with numbers—and a digital one. Or even a combination—an analog face with a digital inset. I have an analog watch that I've found I wear quite often for workouts that I'm not trying to time super-accurately (say, down to the seconds). It has a rotating bezel or ring around the exterior of the face, numbered from 0 to 60. I rotate the 0 mark to wherever the minute hand is when I start my walk. When I finish my walk, the minute hand then shows how long I've walked on the numbered bezel.

If that low-tech approach doesn't do it for you, here are some of the features you can look for in a digital watch, listed in my subjective order of importance:

1. **Stopwatch feature.** This is the simplest way to time your workouts. Look for one that can display the time of day on the face even while the stopwatch is running—it's convenient not to have to switch back and forth.

2. **Alarm clock.** You'll never have an excuse to miss an early-morning walk, even when away from home, if your watch has a reliable and easy-to-use alarm clock.

3. **Countdown timer.** Great for some of the workouts described in this chapter. Say you want to walk hard in one direction for 20 minutes before turning back; you can set the timer to alert you when 20 minutes is up. It's also handy for timing stuff around the kitchen, or enforcement with the kids ("Just 10 more minutes of *Toy Story*, then it's up to bed—I'm setting the watch!").

4. **Light.** It may seem like overkill, but if you know you'll be doing early-morning or evening walks in winter, it's helpful when checking your start and finish times.

5. **Split timer.** This calculates intermediate times while the stopwatch is running. For example, if you're doing laps around a track and want to know your time for each mile, you'd hit the split button as you finish every fourth lap. It would show the elapsed time since the last split—in other words, your time for just that mile.

6. **Memory.** If you want to not only know your splits but also record them in your training log, get a watch with a memory that allows you to display your splits later.

The bad news is that this calculation can be pretty inaccurate. Especially if, for example, you're more or less fit or active or heavy than the average person. A far more accurate way to determine your maximum heart rate is with an actual fitness test or stress test on a treadmill, administered by your doctor or another qualified professional; some fitness centers and most exercise science labs have the capacity to give you a test like this. So if you're serious about using a heart-rate monitor, consider such a test. Otherwise, stick with the age-based estimate.

Here are some exercise heart-rate zones for walking workouts, corresponding to the activity pyramid.

	Goal	Target Heart Rate (% of maximum)	Typical Speeds
Fast walks	Build speed and total fitness	75 to 90%	More than 4.5 mph
Longer walks (45 to 60 minutes)	Burn calories, control weight	65 to 75%	3.5 to 4.5 mph
Moderate daily 30-minute walks	Improve health, feel better	55 to 65%	3 to 4 mph

Here's an example. Edna is a 42-year-old woman, and she wants to know her target heart rate for a 45- to 60-minute walk at level 2 (weight loss) on the activity pyramid. First she estimates her maximum heart rate: 226 – 42 = 184 beats per minute. Now she calculates 65 and 75 percent of that, by multiplying by 0.65 and 0.75:

0.65 x 184 = 120
0.75 x 184 = 138

So Edna's target heart-rate range for her workout is between 120 and 138 beats per minute. If she's going only 45 minutes, she might push toward the upper end of the range; if she'll go an hour or more, she could err toward the lower end. She might also stay closer to 120 beats per minute if she's not feeling great today, or it's extra hot, or there are other stresses in her life. You should never become fixated on a specific heart rate—just use it as a guide. It's still most important to listen to your body and how it feels.

Using a heart-rate monitor

You can measure your heart rate the old-fashioned way, by simply placing your fingers lightly on your carotid artery on either side of your throat. This can give a fairly accurate measurement—just count for 10 seconds and multiply by 6 to get the beats per minute—and it's pretty easy to find your pulse when you're exercising. But you generally have to stop what you're doing to get your pulse, which is no bargain if you're trying to maintain your heart rate in a certain range during a continuous workout.

It's simpler and faster to wear a heart-rate monitor. The best consist of two parts. The monitor itself is a strap that's worn around the chest, with two leads (just flat plastic areas) that rest below the breasts or pectoral muscles. Some sports bras are made to hold a monitor in the bottom across the front. The heart-rate signal is transmitted to a wrist receiver unit, which looks like a slightly oversize digital watch. It displays your heart rate at the moment, in beats per minute, along with other information that you might use during your workout.

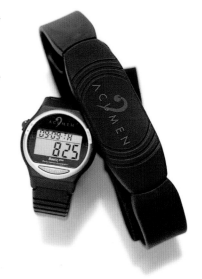

Picking a monitor

Heart-rate monitors offer a variety of functions related to measuring, reporting, and recording your heart rate while exercising. Some also include many of the features that you find in a good digital watch. Most people don't need all the bells and whistles, and given that monitors start at less than $75—but it's possible to spend well over twice that—it's worth thinking carefully about which features you will and won't use. Here's my prioritized list of some of the features; I consider only the first two essential.

1. **Stopwatch feature.** It's convenient to be able to glance at both your heart rate and your exercise time on one device.

Walk Talk: Can a heart-rate monitor tell me if I'm getting in better shape?

Your heart rate during exercise and during the recovery right afterward is an ideal indicator of your fitness level. Here are three tests you can do every once in a while (say, every three weeks) to quantify your improvements—and they also make for great workouts themselves:

1. **Hold that heart rate.** Stroll easily for 5 minutes to warm up, then head out for a walk on one of your standard courses that normally takes 20 to 40 minutes. Choose a heart rate that you consider challenging but in control (about a 7 RPE), and then stay within three beats of that heart rate for the whole walk. (If you're not sure, consider a heart rate in the typical range for your age.) Then accurately time how long it takes to cover your course. In a few weeks walk the same course holding the *same heart rate*. As your fitness improves, you should be able to walk faster, and finish the course faster, at the same effort level. That shows an increase in your cardiorespiratory efficiency.

2. **Match your time.** After an easy 10-minute warm-up at the track, tackle walking a mile at a pace that you know will be hard, but that you can just manage. Walk with an even tempo—if your goal is 14 minutes, walk each lap as close to 3:30 (3 minutes 30 seconds) as possible. Then measure your heart rate immediately after you finish the mile.

In five or six weeks repeat the test, walking a mile at the same speed. As your fitness improves, your heart rate will be lower even as you maintain the same pace. You'll probably notice that you're not breathing as hard or feeling as challenged, either.

3. **Check your recovery.** After either of these tests, continue to watch your heart rate. Accurately note how long it takes (from the moment you stopped walking fast) for your heart rate to drop below 110 beats per minute, and then below 100 beats per minute. As your fitness improves, you'll see your heart rate drop more rapidly, and your recovery time to these two benchmarks will shorten. The faster your recovery, the better your overall fitness.

Approximate Age	Target Heart Rate (65 to 75% of max) (beats per minute)
20 to 30	130 to 155
30 to 40	125 to 150
40 to 50	115 to 140
50 and above	110 to 130

Time for 1 Mile (4 laps) (minutes)	Time for 0.25 Mile (1 lap) (minutes:seconds)
20	5:00
18	4:30
16	4:00
15	3:45
14	3:30
13	3:15
12	3:00
11	2:45
10	2:30
9	2:15
8	2:00

2. **Set a target range, with alarm.** This allows you to enter the upper and lower limits for your target heart rate (120 and 138 beats per minute in the previous example). On some models you can set both a visual signal (say, a flashing star) and an audible one (beep) when you go out of range.

3. **Accumulated time in and out of range.** If you want to know exactly how much of your workout you spent in the target heart-rate range, you'll need this.

4. **Memory.** Some monitors just recall your workout time and how much time you spent in target range. Others can play back your minute-by-minute measurements, so that you can see, for example, how your heart rate climbed during each speedy interval and dropped as you eased up to recover.

5. **Download to a computer.** Why have detailed playback of your workout if you can't store it in your computer, enter it in your digital training log, and print out the heart-rate highlights? Well, you can with the interface cables and software made by some manufacturers.

My verdict on heart-rate monitors

A heart-rate monitor is an accurate way to get feedback on your workout intensity, and I think they can be invaluable for serious athletes in training. I've used them regularly myself and with athletes I coach. Monitors can also be an effective motivational tool. I got one for my sister-in-law one Christmas and—testament to what a great sister-in-law she is—she's said she really likes it. But I actually believe her. She's a fairly consistent exerciser, but she hadn't felt she wasn't getting enough out of her workouts. Wearing the monitor helped her realize that she really hadn't been challenging herself. Cruising along on the treadmill reading the paper wasn't enough—she really had to push herself once in a while, and the monitor helped.

But I also find that once people wear a monitor for a while, they begin to recognize when they're working and when they're not just by how it feels. That Rate of Perceived Exertion stuff isn't malarkey—we really can sense our effort level fairly reliably, especially with experience. Do you still need a heart-rate monitor for every workout then? Probably not. But it might still be useful for a couple of key workouts a month, or to check up on yourself and see if your fitness is improving.

The bottom line is that if you're a gadget geek, this is the ultimate flexible exercise gadget. You can wear it during practically any activity, and it's very informative. But if you're not into hard-

Heart-Rate Monitors	
PROS	**CONS**
Most accurate indicator of effort level while working out.	Depends on an accurate measure of your maximum heart rate to truly be effective.
Easy to use, can provide audible signal when you go out of range.	The audible signal can drive you (and whomever you're walking with) crazy.
Fancy ones can be used with high-tech treadmills to actually adjust the machine's speed to keep you in target range.	Heart rate can be influenced by heat, dehydration, or other stress.
Can be a good motivational tool.	Can be another gadget that sits on the shelf.

ware, don't waste your time; a monitor will only frustrate you, and there are viable low-tech alternatives (such as RPE and counting your steps) to help you keep your walking intensity on track.

Walk Talk: For really fast walking, do I need running shoes?

Read my lips: *Even if you walk fast, you do not need to wear running shoes.* There are plenty of walking shoes available that are made with the same lightweight and durable materials as high-quality running shoes, but on a sole that's better designed for walking. The key is finding these shoes—they may not be the first walking shoes you see in the store, and they certainly won't be the only ones.

Many manufacturers still make lots of their walking shoes with mostly or entirely leather uppers. And they're typically—surprise!—all white. Manufacturers defend this utter lack of creativity with the argument that it's what walkers are asking for. But I think it's mostly because in many retail stores the salespeople sell all-leather, all-white shoes for walking around and casual wear, and *running* shoes for serious fitness walking.

The heavier all-leather shoes are usually fine for moderate-paced walking. But as you speed up and really turn your walk into a workout, you need lighter weight, more flexibility, and greater breathability than many all-leather shoes can provide. Fortunately, most manufacturers make at least one or two models that are truly designed for fast walking, with the following features:
• A very rounded or beveled heel.
• Great flexibility at the ball of the foot, but support through the arch.
• Some lightweight mesh materials in the upper for both breathability and weight reduction.
• Durable cushioning materials in the midsole, which will help the shoe keep absorbing shock all the way through its three- to five-month life.

So how do you battle the forces that are trying to get you into running shoes and find quality walking shoes for high-speed walking? Here are four things you can do:

1. Know what you're looking for. When you go to the store, already know some quality athletic walking shoe models. Several places to learn what's out there are regular athletic shoe reviews in *Health Magazine*, and manufacturers' Web sites (see Footwear in the resource section).

2. Support stores that carry what you want. Sometimes specialty running or athletic stores have a decent offering for serious walkers. They understand that athletes come in all shapes and sizes, and some walk and some run. If you find such a store, reward them for carrying good walking shoes by buying there—it's worth it.

3. Scold stores that don't have what you want. Don't buy a running shoe just because a 19-year-old salesperson says it's the same as a walking shoe. If they don't have what you're looking for, don't buy there. And let them know why.

4. Consider shopping online. Trying on shoes is best, but if you don't have a store that meets your needs in your area, or you think you know what size you take in the model you want to buy, consider the Web. A growing array of models is available online. See "Footwear" in the resource list at the end of this book to learn more about walking manufacturers and shoes.

Since it's the one piece of gear you really need, it's worth some effort to find a pair that really works for you. Remember, how a shoe feels on your foot is the most important thing.

15

Total Fitness: Weights and Cross-Training

Building a harder body

If you're interested in complete fitness, you'll need a strength-training program designed to get you there. This means an increased focus on total-body movements, not just exercises that isolate one muscle or group. For example, many beginning programs (such as the one in chapter 10) have you do triceps extensions, focused on strengthening the back of the upper arm. In this routine you'll do dips instead. They give the triceps a great workout, but they also challenge the shoulders and upper back, require the abdominals to hold proper body position, and demand coordination of the entire body to maintain balance during the movement.

Another reason to move into this routine is that change is critical to improving your strength. Do the same exercises indefinitely and your muscles become accustomed to them. The exercises become less of a challenge and won't improve your strength nearly as much.

Lift right (then left)

A key to successful weight lifting is good technique. One of the most common errors I see is people moving the weights too fast and letting momentum, not their muscles, do the work. Here are some tips for success:

• Concentrate on slow, controlled movements—don't let momentum do the work for you—and move your joints through their full range of motion. Some coaches recommend taking 2 counts on the up (or working) movement and 4 counts on the down (or recovery).

• When possible, exhale while lifting the weight, and inhale on the recovery or between reps.

• Maintain good posture. Focus on stabilizing your body throughout all movements with your abdominal and back muscles.

• Lifting shouldn't hurt, but it should be hard. Select a weight so that you are just able to finish the designated number of repetitions on the last set but would be hard pressed to do more.

• Keep progressing; this is critical to long-term success. If you don't want your strength to plateau, you have to keep challenging your muscles. When a weight becomes easy to lift, add more. Increase to the next weight (usually a three-to five-pound increase) and reduce the number of repetitions if necessary, until you're able to build up to the full target number again.

- Vary your routine. Like increasing the weight, changing some of your exercises every 8 to 16 weeks alters muscle loads and movements and enhances the benefits.

The total-body routine

This program is fairly challenging. It assumes you've been doing some resistance training already (for example, the equivalent of at least 8 to 12 weeks' worth of the program shown in chapter 10) and have a base level of fitness. You also should be familiar with weights and confident using them.

This is an at-home routine—you'll need a weight bar and weights or dumbbells of various sizes (probably 5 to 25 pounds, depending on your fitness), a floor mat, a bench or chair, and a chin-up bar (for example, the kind suspended in a doorway). Equivalent exercises can also be done with machines at a gym.

Do 12 repetitions of an exercise; rest, then do a second set of 12 repetitions, unless otherwise noted. Select a weight so that you can just barely finish the second set of 12. Do the routine two or three times a week; the ideal is five workouts every two weeks. Do the exercises in the order described, to work paired muscle groups.

1. **Push-ups.** Begin with only your knees and hands on the floor, knees together, hands shoulder-width apart, arms straight. Keep your back flat and your head level. Bend your arms and lower your chest to the floor, then press your arms out straight and return to the starting position.

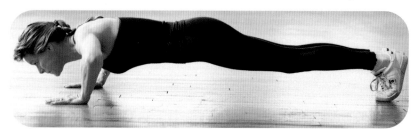

When you're able to finish 10 reps, go to full push-ups, with only your toes and hands on the ground and your body held board-flat from shoulders to toes.

2. **Bent-over rows.** Lean forward with your left foot on the ground and your right knee and hand on a chair or bench. Your chest should be facing the ground; your left hand holds the weight and hangs straight down toward the floor. Pull the weight up to your chest and squeeze your shoulder blades together to finish; then lower the weight slowly.

3. **Lunge with bar or weights.** Start by holding a dumbbell in each hand at your sides, with both feet together; take a large step forward. Bend your forward knee (maintain a tall posture; don't push your bending knee beyond your foot) to extend your back leg, then press forcefully off your forward leg to return to standing. Do 10 reps on each leg, alternating.

4. **Full abdominal crunch.** Lying on your back with your arms and legs both pointed toward the ceiling, tighten your abdominals to lift both shoulders and hips off the mat; attempt to extend both feet and hands toward the ceiling. Hold momentarily, then relax. Begin with 10 reps and build to 20.

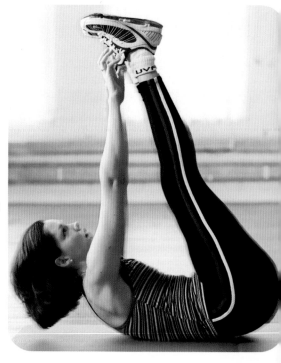

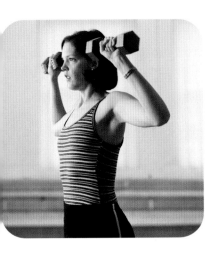

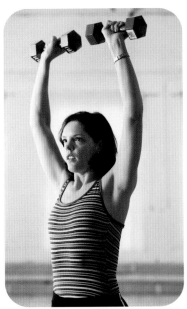

5. Overhead press. Stand with your feet shoulder-width apart, knees slightly bent. Hold weight(s) in your hands beside your shoulders. (If you're using a single bar, it should rest across the top of your chest.) Slowly extend your arms straight up overhead, without locking your elbows, then bend your elbows and return to the starting position.

6. Pull-ups (or assisted pull-ups). Hang from a horizontal bar, arms extended, palms forward, your hand grip slightly wider than shoulder-width; slowly pull your chin up to the bar, then slowly lower yourself. If needed, get a little help until you can do these alone (or bend your legs and rest your toes on a bench to help somewhat).

An easier option is to suspend a broomstick securely between two identical-height chairs. Lying on your back between the chairs, reach up and hold the broomstick with your hands slightly more than shoulder-width apart. Slowly pull your upper body off the ground until the top of your chest reaches the stick; slowly return to the starting position. (In the gym you can use a lat pull-down machine.)

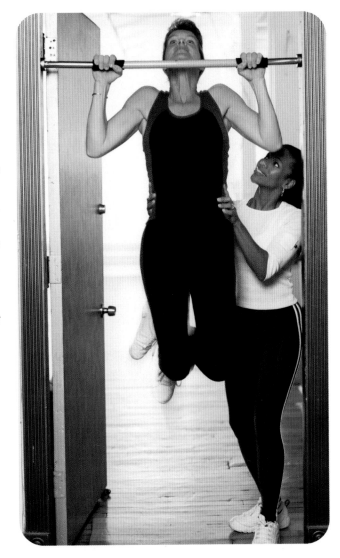

7. Squat with bar or weights. Stand tall with your feet hip-width apart, and place a weight bar across your shoulders (wrap with a towel for comfort) or hold dumbbells at your sides. Bend your knees and hips to drop to a half-sitting position, keeping your upper body as erect as possible, then stand back up.

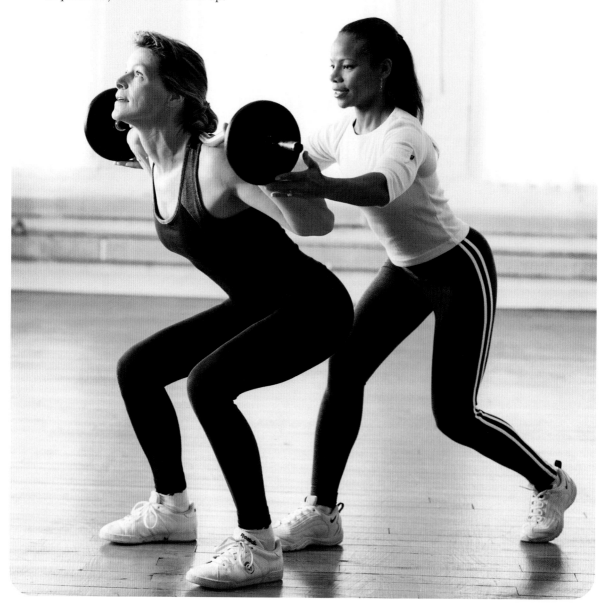

8. Isometric side support. Lie on your right side on an exercise mat. Place your right forearm on the ground below your right shoulder, thus lifting your upper body off the mat. Straighten your body so that it's supported between your right forearm and foot, with the right side of your body facing the floor and your left side facing the ceiling. Hold for 15 seconds. Build up to 30 seconds. Do twice on each side.

If this is too difficult, begin with your knees bent and suspend your body between your right arm and knee.

9. Dips. Sit on the edge of a bench with your hands on the edge next to your buttocks. Slide your butt forward off the edge, bend your arms and drop until your elbows are bent almost 90 degrees, then press back up. Keeping your feet on the ground with your legs bent makes these easier; having your feet on the ground with your legs straight forward is harder; elevating your feet on another chair or bench is hardest.

To really challenge yourself, hold your full body weight between two parallel bars with your body upright and your legs hanging down; bend your arms and lower your body until your elbows are bent almost 90 degrees, then press back up.

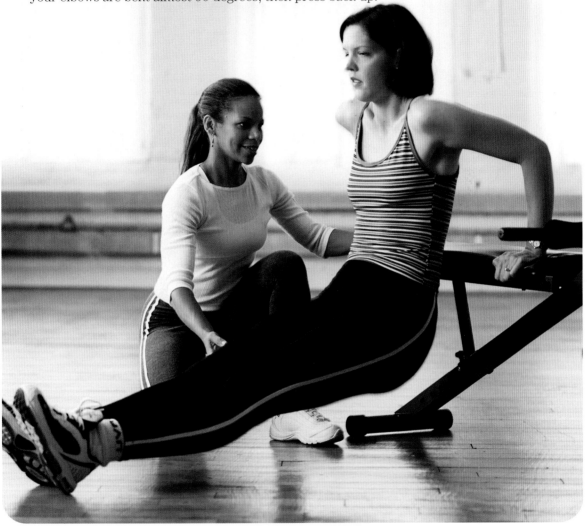

10. Biceps curl (both arms simultaneously). Stand with your feet shoulder-width apart and your knees slightly bent. Hold a bar or dumbbell in front of your thighs with your palms forward and your arms fully extended. Bend your elbows to slowly bring the weight(s) up in front of your shoulders, then slowly lower them. Keep the weights level—parallel with the ground—throughout this motion.

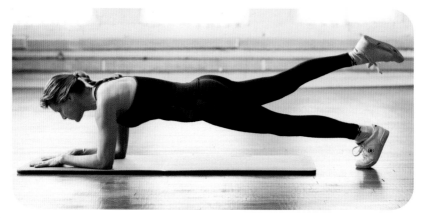

11. **Modified plank.** Lie flat on the floor, facedown. Keeping your body flat, lift your body entirely off the floor, supporting your torso on your elbows and forearms, and your legs on your toes; only your forearms and toes should touch the ground. (Your abdominal muscles will be working to hold this position.) Slowly raise your right leg 6 to 10 inches, hold for a 2-count, and lower. Alternate lifting legs, 10 on each side. As your fitness improves, hold the leg up for a 5-count.

Building total fitness

The human body is capable of an immense variety of things. Some are impressive to the point of being almost unbelievable. Top weight lifters can heft several times their own body weights. Dancers appear to float in the air, and gymnasts can bend and balance in ways that I find unimaginable. The skills of athletes in so many sports, from the ball-and-stick games like baseball and tennis to pure athletics such as the high jump or throwing the javelin, never cease to amaze me.

Even though you may never aspire to these heights, such variety in athletic prowess is a reminder that to be completely fit means more than just being a certain weight, or even being able to walk so far in a certain amount of time. True fitness has lots of facets, and even if you'll never try to run a four-minute mile or do a triple axel in figure skating, it's worth challenging and im-

Walk Talk: I don't have time after my walking workout to do my weight lifting all at once. Do I have to get up earlier or could I split up the weight program on separate days?

First of all, plan on getting up earlier only if you know it will last. If you think you're likely to skip workouts, it's not worth the risk. But the idea of breaking the program into two parts is great. The basic goal is to exercise most of the major muscle groups at least two days per week; doing some muscles on Monday and Thursday, and others on Tuesday and Friday, for example, is fine. Just try to work paired muscles (for example, the chest and back) on the same day.

The program here could break up like this:

Routine 1. Push-ups, bent-over rows, lunges, abdominal crunch, overhead press, pull-ups.

Routine 2. Squats, isometric side support, dips, biceps curl, modified plank, abdominal crunch.

Then do a weight workout at least four times each week, alternating routines 1 and 2. And yes, abdominal crunches are important enough to do with every workout.

proving all these facets. True fitness assures you that your body will always be ready for any adventures or dangers—including illness—that life might throw your way. This is central to living life to its fullest—the physical confidence to always be willing and able to try something new. Here are the basic elements of overall fitness.

Endurance

Stamina or endurance is the body's ability to continuously maintain a certain level of effort. It reflects both the intensity of an activity (say, walking at 4 miles per hour), and how long you can sustain it (such as doing it for 8 miles nonstop). But in endurance training the emphasis is usually on duration, while the intensity is more modest.

Why Do You Want It?

Endurance is critical to success in continuous sports and activities ranging from soccer games and road races to an all-day hike. But it also helps in daily life. Sustained low-intensity activities are easier if you have greater endurance; muscular endurance can be beneficial even for something as simple as maintaining good posture when you have to stand for long periods.

Speed

I'm talking about the kind of speed reflected by how fast your body can do a repetitive movement, like walking, for a fairly short time. (That's different from what some coaches might call "quickness"—the ability to change directions quickly, needed in sports such as fencing and basketball.) How fast you can walk 0.5 to 1 mile, for example, is reflective of your speed. It's limited by both your technique and your body's ability to utilize energy very rapidly.

Why Do You Want It?

Sure, increasing your speed will improve your 1-mile walking time, but that's sort of an esoteric goal if you're not a competitor. Still, the faster your maximum speed, the easier your slightly-less-than-maximum efforts become. If you can walk 1 mile in 12 minutes (a 5-mile-per-hour pace), then walking 3 miles in 42 minutes (a swift 14-minute-per-mile pace) gets a lot easier. Physiologically, you're building your body's high-intensity energy systems with speed. And there's a weight-loss benefit: You're creating lots of energy-burning capacity in your muscle cells, which helps make them better calories burners all the time.

Strength

Stated in simplest form, the greatest amount of force a muscle can generate represents its strength. But there's an endurance component to strength, too: how many times you can lift a weight (for instance) that's less than your maximum. Strength isn't just related to muscle size—it's also related to how many of a muscle's fibers you're able to effectively use in a given movement, a factor that improves with training.

Why Do You Want It?

Increasing your muscular strength is central to increasing the strength of your bones. Stronger muscles, through both exercise and routine daily movements, stimulate your bones to maintain a higher, healthier density and stave off osteoporosis. But there are mundane reasons why strength is good, too—the ability to lift and carry things in daily life, or to simply get up from sitting on the floor. Self-image and self-satisfaction are also valid benefits: Stronger muscles are firmer, and shapelier, and they'll probably help you feel better about yourself.

Flexibility

How much you're able to move at your joints is called your range of motion. This range is limited first by the structure of your bones and how they connect. But the stiffness of the softer tissues around the joints is important, too. Muscles, tendons, and ligaments all affect your range of motion, and here's the rub: These soft tissues all tend to lose some of their elasticity with age. Muscles can also tighten as they're exercised and become stronger. So the core measure of flexibility is how much of your range of motion you're able to maintain throughout your body's joints.

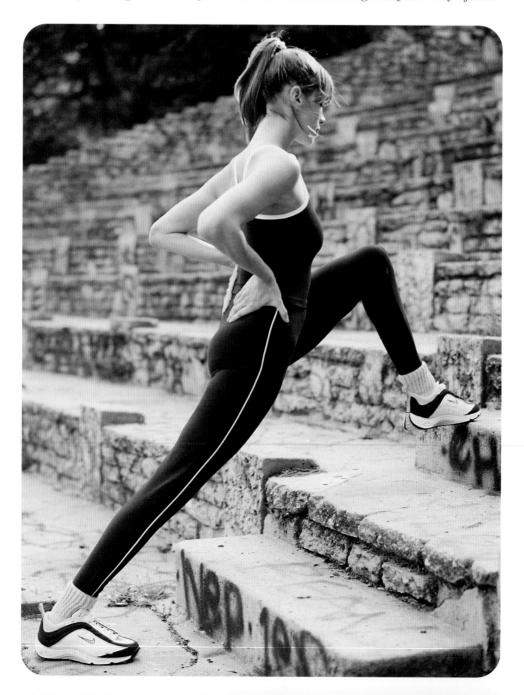

Why Do You Want It?

Flexibility is truly a measure of your functionality. More flexible muscles appear less likely to be injured. The chance of chronic problems such as soreness, and acute ones like muscle pulls or strains, both appear to be lower in people who've maintained a healthy range of motion. Performance in most sports is also enhanced by greater flexibility. But even routine movements, from getting out of a car to picking something up off the floor, are easier and more comfortable if you've maintained your full range of motion. The trick isn't trying to become super-flexible; it's maintaining enough of your natural range of movement to be functional and healthy.

Balance and coordination

This is a broad category, and in some ways it reflects other elements of fitness combined: Strength, flexibility, speed, and endurance all play a role in your ability to make controlled movements, maintain your balance, and have your body do what you request of it. But coordination and balance are also something more. Your body's ability to swiftly process information and respond—where your limbs are, how fast you're moving, whether you're falling or not—reflects your level of coordination. Many of these things aren't done consciously, but happen almost instantaneously at a neuromuscular level.

Why Do You Want It?

Differences in balance and coordination are why one person can balance on one leg and juggle while another has trouble just standing still on two feet with his eyes closed. But both have far-reaching implications not just for parlor tricks and sports but also for lifelong well-being. Being co-ordinated enough to try a wide variety of physical activities is one of the keys to keeping yourself interested in exercise and moving for a lifetime. It also means you're less likely to suffer injuries and falls, and more likely to catch and correct yourself if you do.

Pick your cross-training

Vanity, health, and longevity are all great reasons to be fit, but the best of all, I think, is that being fit lets you use your body in all kinds of new ways. Competitive athletes call it cross-training; they use other sports to get better at theirs. I think trying other sports is an end in itself. Of course, cross-training makes you even fitter, so you can try even more things with confidence. And what goes around comes around: If you try a variety of activities, you'll ultimately be a better walker, as well as stronger, faster, more flexible, and better coordinated.

Pick your cross-training based on these three criteria, in order of importance:

1. **You enjoy it.** If it's not fun, you're not going to make something a regular part of your weekly routine.
2. **You can do it fairly easily.** It's terrific if you enjoy speed skating and find it a great alternative workout—unless you've moved to southern New Mexico, far from indoor ice rinks. Pick activities that don't create extra barriers to participation. Exercise is hard enough as it is.
3. **It challenges a lot of the elements of fitness.** Taking an intense step or kickboxing class at the gym is good, because it will work on some of your endurance, speed, strength, and coordination. Just grinding away on a stair climber, on the other hand, offers only endurance and modest strength work.

There are too many different sports, games, and recreational pursuits to possibly create a comprehensive list of good choices. Instead, here are a variety of activities with a mention of the unique benefits they offer or fitness elements they build, and some comments on my personal favorites. (Hey, it's my book—I can do that.) And remember that you should always give yourself credit in your exercise log for time you spend doing physical activities other than walking. Your cross-training can even replace the walking (or strength or flexibility work) it most closely resembles as far as the intensity and time you spend.

Have fun with cross-training

1. **Running, including jogging, road racing, cross-country and trail running.** Let's get one thing clear, just in case I haven't been explicit enough already: You don't have to graduate from walking to running to get *really* fit or become a *real* athlete. If you learn nothing else in this book, I hope it's perfectly obvious that it's possible to walk far enough and fast enough (and to use such things as terrain and Nordic walking poles) to get a tremendous workout and burn just as many calories in walking as in running. However, it's also likely that you'll never walk as fast as you can run because of a simple biomechanical truth—in running your legs act like alternating springs, pushing you into the air with each stride, then coiling (actually bending) as you hit the ground, before bouncing into the air for the next step. Thus they store a bit of energy then give it back on each stride, which makes for greater speed than walking.

   The downside of all that energy storing and rebounding is the physical shock you experience with each step. In running you strike the ground with a force of two to four times your body weight or more on each step; the less skilled a runner you are, the higher that impact tends to be. Research shows that that has the benefit of providing good stimulus for bone density, but can also lead to impact related injuries such as stress fractures. In walking, by comparison, impact loads range from one to one-and-a-half times body weight, even for high speed competitive racewalkers.

   So why do I still sprinkle some occasional running into my routine? Because I was a cross-country runner in high school and I still enjoy occasionally running on trails and in parkland, especially on softer more-forgiving surfaces. There are times when I just want to cover more ground in less time, and for that running can't be beat. Just be extra sure you wear high-quality running shoes appropriate for your foot type.

   What running offers:
   - You'll always be able to go farther running than walking for a given amount of time.
   - Running is a terrific workout for the legs and can develop a plyometric strength (think springiness) that you simply won't get from walking.
   - Running is a tremendous aerobic conditioner; longer slow runs build endurance, while shorter, faster runs boost speed and high intensity (anaerobic) fitness.

2. **Swimming, including water running and walking and water aerobics classes.** I've always enjoyed the water. But it was during recovery from surgery as an adult that I realized the true power of the activity. It can be a phenomenal total-body workout, yet offers almost no risk of impact related injuries. In fact it is often the conditioner of choice for runners or walkers who've had stress fractures, knee surgeries, or other injuries. For those who don't

swim, or who want to more fully mimic the running or walking motion during rehabilitation, you can wear a flotation vest that supports your body upright in the water, allowing you to walk or run in water that's over your head.

Swimming is a perfect complement to walking because the emphasis tends to be reversed—more challenge to the upper body in swimming, more to the lower in walking, and great work for the torso in both. One way to improve the balance is to mix up your strokes. Don't just do the freestyle (crawl), but also do some breaststrokes (great for legs and hips), backstrokes (for powerful shoulders), kicks for the legs with the kickboard, and then pull a pull-buoy for the arms. It's a versatile activity that can offer a challenge for any fitness level.

What swimming offers:

- Low impact; great strength workout for shoulders, chest, and upper back.
- Easy sustained swimming gives similar endurance benefits to longer walks.
- Add speedy intervals and you can boost the heart rate and equal the intensity of the fastest speed workout or hill climb.

Looking for similar benefits but not comfortable in water over your head? Consider a water aerobics class where you stand or walk in chest-deep water, thus keeping impact negligible but getting the dynamic resistance of water during your movements, and a commensurately intense workout.

3. **Paddle Sports, including canoeing, kayaking, and surfing.** Years ago a friend introduced me to white-water kayaking—knowing that I'd been a flat-water canoeist since my youth. I practiced for sodden but joyful hours on a nearby pond. But the biggest surprise was what a total-body workout paddling is. Done correctly, the legs work hard to connect your body to the boat and transfer the power of your strokes to the hull. The torso has to be a sort of universal joint, connecting the paddling upper body to the legs, which control the attitude of the boat (or, in surfing, the board). And in white-water kayaking it all has to work together flawlessly if (or in my case, *when*) you tip over and have to Eskimo roll upright.

There are too many variations of paddle craft to describe here, from the old standard aluminum canoe to sleek fiberglass sea kayaks that knife gracefully through ocean waves. But it's worth noting that kayaks in particular come in three broad varieties: 1) longer, pointier sea kayaks designed for efficiency when ocean paddling; 2) shorter, stubbier white-water kayaks, which are highly maneuverable for negotiating rocky rivers; and 3) a wide range of recreational kayaks for general flat-water rivers, lakes, and calm ocean conditions. This last group has opened the world of kayaking to just about everyone, as the boats are broad and stable in the water, easy to master, and reasonably priced; you can get a starter setup with boat, paddle, and personal flotation device (a fancy name for a life vest) for under $500.

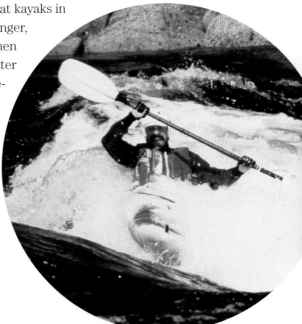

What paddling offers:

- Long, easy paddles build endurance, like moderate to long walks.
- Vigorous paddling is solid strength training for arms, shoulders, chest, back, and abdomen.
- Balance and controlling body position become second nature over time.
- You can choose an environment that mirrors your mood (and risk aversion).
- Surfing waves or paddling white water is much like an interval workout, with high intensity efforts followed by easier recoveries.

4. **Court Sports, including volleyball, basketball, tennis, racquetball, handball, squash, and badminton.** These sports offer a tremendous range of options, from team activities such as volleyball and basketball to one-on-one sports such as tennis or squash. In most cases the intensity and quality of the workout depends on your skill level. After all, it's hard to work up much of a sweat in tennis if you aren't able to return a shot and spend most of your time picking up missed balls (although you can still get in a good bit of walking). The workout also depends greatly on how seriously you're playing. For example, volleyball comes in many varieties, from the backyard brand played with a hot dog in one hand, to an organized six-on-six indoor game or intense two-on-two beach volleyball match.

Most court sports alternate high- and low-intensity periods; a flurry of movement during a rally in tennis or volleyball, say, alternating with the brief respite as you set up for the next service. They'll also build leg strength; just think of the tensed muscles of the "ready" position with your weight on the balls of your feet—and quickness and agility to get to the ball. In general, there's a good mix of upper- and lower-body exercise in this family of activities.

What court sports offer:

- All provide some upper-body work and eye-hand coordination, either to handle or strike a ball, or to use a racquet.
- Some require a good deal of running on the court, which can build stamina.
- Serious play requires quick lateral (sideward) and backward movements, all of which work your muscles very differently than walking.
- In more vigorous play your agility will be enhanced by the need to react quickly to the ball (or shuttlecock); these sports can do lots for balance and coordination.

Looking for similar benefits off the court? Try fitness classes such as dance, aerobics, or step class, especially those with bounding or jumping, lateral and upper-body movements.

5. **Field sports, including soccer, lacrosse, field hockey, rugby and football, as well as baseball and softball.** There are what I call "flowing" field sports such as soccer and field hockey, and the more stop-and-go games of softball and baseball where all players but the hitter are sitting on the bench or standing in the field. It's fair to say that the flow sports tend to be more intense exercise, but like so many sports, the quality of the workout depends directly on how seriously you're playing. Just kicking the soccer ball around the backyard may not be much effort, but playing a real game on a full field is certain get your heart rate up fast!

What field sports offer:

- A challenging combination of quickness and sprints, for example as you burst for the ball or a breakaway, and more sustained lower-intensity movement during the regular flow of the game.

- Many field sports will require swift lateral and even backward movements, especially when your team is on defense; add to that the need to be aware of where you are on the field.

- The non-flow sports—baseball and softball—won't build as much aerobic endurance, but will have short bursts of high intensity activity, and are sure to develop eye-hand coordination if you work on your hitting and fielding skills.

6. **Bicycling, including recreational, road, and mountain biking.** I'd always ridden a traditional road bicycle—skinnier tires, curved racing handlebars, and painful seat. But when my son was born I'd avoided putting on a bike seat for him, given how skittish the bike seemed and fearing that I wouldn't be stable enough with him on board. Then my wife and I went to Nantucket and rented some hybrid bikes, with the lower, more stable frames, slightly thicker tires, upright handlebars and vastly more comfortable seats borrowed from mountain bikes.

For my next birthday, what did I get but a shiny new mountain bike . . . with a child seat attached! My infant son and daughter logged many miles on board, then graduated to a bike trailer, then a tag-along (a trailing bike wheel with handlebars, seat, and pedals that really drive the wheel), before riding themselves. All of which is a testament to the amazing improvements in bicycling gear and convenience over the years. You can select a high-performance, super-light, skinny-tired road-racing bike; a slightly beefier touring bike for commuting or recreational riding; a mountain bike with thick, knobby tires and shock absorbers for grinding up and bouncing down hillsides; and now a host of hybrids with cushiony seats, upright handlebar configurations, tires of various sizes and textures, and myriad frame shapes. For example, I bought my mother a step-through frame that's just as it sounds—slung low so you don't have to swing a leg over to climb aboard, but can simply step across in front of the seat. There are even recumbent bikes that allow you to lean back on a chair-like seat and push pedals out in front of you, ideal for folks with lower back troubles.

The bottom line is that there is a bicycle for absolutely any age or ability, and just about any terrain. Furthermore, in a world where gas prices will only keep rising and global warming is a real and recognized threat, a bicycle can be much more than exercise—it can be a great way to get around and save the planet at the same time!

Amy Dawson's 30th birthday was upon her, and she was not about to pass into her fourth decade quietly. She knew exactly how she wanted to feel: "Like the queen of the world and mistress of all I surveyed." Where did Amy figure she could get such feeling? A Caribbean cruise? A luxurious spa getaway? Walking a marathon?

Wait a second—a marathon? You betcha. That's exactly how you're going to feel, at least according to a first-time finisher in the Portland Marathon walking division whose story Amy had read about in *WALKING* Magazine. A chemical engineer at Procter and Gamble in Cincinnati, Amy snagged her two walking buddies, twins Karen McCann and Kimberly Kent, and recruited them to train with her for the January 2000 Walt Disney World Marathon.

The Turning Point

None of the women had ever imagined she could walk a marathon. As fitness walkers, 7 to 10 miles a week seemed to do it. Besides being so busy with their jobs (Karen and Kimberly are social workers), Kim's wedding was looming and Karen was to be her maid of honor. Amy was deeply involved in planning the big affair. Nevertheless, they all were drawn to the 18-week training program in the *WALKING* Magazine article. Unlike so many marathon programs, it didn't require endless weekend walks. This seemed too good to be true: a series of six critical long weekend walks on alternate weeks, and shorter but speedier midweek workouts. (See chapter 19 for the program.)

A Week in Their Lives

After Amy printed out color calendars of the training program for each of them, she figured out loops that they could use for their long weekend walks; friends have since asked for copies. Although the women did their midweek walks alone, they spoke and e-mailed daily to encourage and push each other.

What bicycling offers:

- In general, a terrific complementary workout to walking that will strengthen the leg muscles with almost no impact.
- An upper-body workout to maintain control and steer the bike; the harder you ride and more hills you climb, the more your arms and torso work.
- Long rides on mild terrain are like endurance walks; bursting up and down hills offers great high-intensity workouts (and plenty of adrenalin rush, if you need that sort of thing).

Looking for similar benefits without hitting the road? Ride a stationary bicycle—there are recumbent models for those with lower-back problems—or try a spinning class.

7. **Snow sports, including cross-country skiing, snowshoeing, downhill skiing, snowboarding, and sledding.** At the Olympic Training Center, they regularly measure the aerobic capacity of athletes by having them run on a treadmill to exhaustion while measuring the amount of oxygen they're utilizing. Distance runners regularly score very highly, as do elite-

Their Biggest Accomplishment

All three finished successfully, with times in the 6:10 to 6:30 range—very impressive, given that the program doesn't promise anything more than breaking 7 hours.

Yet that's not what they consider their biggest accomplishment: It was instead the long workout (two hours and 45 minutes) two weeks before the actual race that fell on Christmas Day. The trio did it in zero-degree weather. Having endured that, no way were they going to be denied their Mickey Mouse medals!

Their Key to Success

When asked by a friend if they were taking any special supplements, they answered, "Blueberry Mickey Mouse waffles!" Every Saturday, Kim's fiancé (now husband), Dave, made brunch for them using his Mickey Mouse waffle iron. As they came in from their long weekend workouts, there were waffles awaiting.

Of course, their team effort was the key. Each had a role—team cheerleader, emotional stabilizer, and organizer/planner.

What's Next?

At the postmarathon breakfast with Dave—he hung Kim's Mickey Mouse medal over the chandelier—they discussed doing the race again. Amy says she definitely will; she couldn't get the smile off her face when she crossed the line, and she's ready to sign up now. Kim is likely to try again, but wants a chance to settle into married life, too. And Karen says probably not yet, because she needs a different type of challenge. So her next goal is to be able to do 10 pull-ups by Labor Day. Hey, this is no Mickey Mouse goal—if she makes it, her husband has promised a weeklong vacation anywhere in the continental United States. No doubt she'll choose a place where she'll feel like the queen of the world and mistress of all she surveys.

level racewalkers, as they've trained their bodies for nonstop aerobic activity. But the very highest scores usually belong to Nordic skiers, because of how they utilize almost all of their muscles from arms and shoulders to torso and legs. Snowshoeing with ski poles gives a similar whole-body workout. Of course it all depends on how hard you work—in Nordic skiing and snowshoeing you can stick with level terrain at the local snow-covered park or golf course, but both become rugged workouts if you seek out hills or venture into the backcountry.

In downhill skiing and snowboarding, a ski lift does the uphill work, but you still get an intense muscular challenge, especially for the thighs and gluteal muscles, as you control your plummet downhill. Of course sledding with the kids flips it around—you get a great workout dragging the toboggan uphill, and get a free ride down.

What snow sports offer:
- A terrific aerobic workout; Nordic skiing and snowshoeing are more consistently intense than downhill, and provide the best total-body conditioning. Done vigorously, they can be among the very best total-body workouts.

- Downhill skiing and snowboarding are great workouts for leg strength and fitness for shorter, more intense bursts of effort.
- All are fun enough to keep you rolling, even as you're working hard; plus they get you outside and keep you active even during winter!

Looking for the benefits without the cold? Consider a Nordic skiing machine or one of the many eccentric training machines in the gym that require simultaneous arm and leg motions.

8. **Ice sports, including speed skating, hockey, figure skating and ice dancing.** Another way to stay active when it gets cold, getting on the ice can also be a great change of pace from walking. Skating is a workout focused on leg strength, but it also obviously builds balance and coordination. Serious hockey can be particularly intense, requiring repeated sprints, total-body strength and coordination with backward skating and abrupt turns and stops. Speed skating demands tremendous power and endurance, particularly for longer events, while figure skating and ice dancing add an artistic element to this great exercise. But even recreational skating on a local pond can be a great balance-builder and overall strength workout for the legs, especially the hips, glutes and thighs.

What ice sports offer:
- Terrific strength workout for the legs, especially thighs and gluteal muscles.
- Will also work the muscles of the torso and will require both strength and flexibility in the back and legs.

Looking for similar benefits on dry land? In-line skating is a terrific workout for thighs and glutes, and can be great fun on paved bike trails; just be sure to wear a helmet and proper pads for your skill level.

9. **Yoga and martial arts.** A common story I hear is of athletes in their forties who discover yoga as the antidote to tightening muscles and stiffening joints resulting from years of endurance or fitness activities. But how do yoga and martial arts fit together? They share the common theme of focusing on the connection between the mind and body, as well as a great emphasis on controlled, deliberate movement. They also require both static (stationary) as well as dynamic (moving) strength and flexibility. Even though I'm not very good at it, I have found yoga to be a phenomenal complement to walking because of the total-body flexibility it encourages. The one limitation is that these don't tend to be self-taught activities; you really need to take instruction to learn them properly.

What yoga and martial arts offer:
- Fantastic body control and flexibility development that really works the entire body.
- Great strength development that over time will lead to long, healthy, toned musculature.
- Truly makes the mind-body connection; you'll find there are many yoga moves you simply aren't going to master without total concentration.

Looking for similar benefits? Consider Pilates, a conditioning program with very challenging isometric and dynamic strength movements, or any of a host of hybrid fitness classes that draw from yoga and martial arts movements.

	Date	Today's Activity Goal(s)	Total Minutes (or √)	Stretch? (√)	Comments, Other Activities? (vigorous chores, sports, other exercise, etc.)	Estimated Miles Walked
Sunday		cross-train				
Monday		1:00, strength				
Tuesday		45				
Wednesday		1:00, speed #6				
Thursday		35				
Friday		off, strength				
Saturday		1:15				

Miles this week: ⎯⎯⎯⎯

Total miles for the year: ⎯⎯⎯⎯

Add a third day of strength training now and then

You'll note that strength workouts are recommended for both Monday and Friday this week. Take a look at speed workout #6 in chapter 14 (see page 156) and you'll see that some strength moves are included there, too. So effectively you're getting strength training three days this week: in the Monday and Friday workouts, plus after Wednesday's speed work. On alternate weeks I'll recommend three strength workouts—an average of five every two weeks—to really help you build overall fitness.

Tip for the week. If you find it hard to get in three strength workouts a week, don't forget the idea of doing a circuit workout (moving quickly through a sequence of exercises 30 seconds at a time) to combine aerobic and strength work. You can also look to your Sunday cross-training as a chance to build strength. Activities such as kayaking, rock climbing, martial arts, and some aerobics classes have plenty of strength training built right into the activity—enough to count as one of your strength days.

	Date	Today's Activity Goal(s)	Total Minutes (or √)	Stretch? (√)	Comments, Other Activities? (vigorous chores, sports, other exercise, etc.)	Estimated Miles Walked
Sunday		cross-train				
Monday		55, strength				
Tuesday		45				
Wednesday		1:00, speed #7				
Thursday		40, strength				
Friday		off				
Saturday		1:30				

Miles this week: _____

Total miles for the year: _____

Try cross-training every week

Cross-training shows up every week now. Hopefully you've discovered activities that you enjoy and have found convenient enough to include regularly. If not, take a look back at chapter 15 for more ideas.

It's also time to sign up for a 10K event in week 48. (See "Events" in the resource list at the back of this book). Check out chapter 16 for ideas on the types of events you might try, and for a pre-event checklist. It's a good reminder of lots of the little things you should do in the days and weeks leading up to your walking event, from making sure you have pins (for pinning your number to your shirt) to checking out your apparel for irritating spots.

Tip for the week. Get a walking partner committed to walking your event with you. Grab your friend an entry form, and even fill it out and send it in if you have to. Then invite your partner to start training with you—the Wednesday speed workouts are especially good to do with someone else, to really get the most out of the effort.

Date	Today's Activity Goal(s)	Total Minutes (or √)	Stretch? (√)	Comments, Other Activities? (vigorous chores, sports, other exercise, etc.)	Estimated Miles Walked
Sunday	cross-train				
Monday	1:00, strength				
Tuesday	45				
Wednesday	1:00, speed #4				
Thursday	45				
Friday	off, strength				
Saturday	1:15				

Miles this week: ——————

Total miles for the year: ——————

Plan the details of your year-end reward

Way back in the beginning of this program I urged you to pick a long-term reward—something big like a hiking vacation in the Rockies or a trip to Europe—if you completed this entire program. Well, the end is in sight, and you have a healthier, stronger, leaner, happier body and mind to show for it. But make sure you're keeping up your end of the deal—you've got a payoff to plan. Hopefully you've been working on it, but if not, get cracking. You deserve it!

Tip for the week. You're doing full-fledged athletic training, with your long and speedy walking workouts, strength training, occasional hikes, and cross-training. This means it's more important than ever to keep up your preventive habits. Daily stretching is crucial, but you may also need the preventive exercise routine shown in chapter 18 (see page 208). Consider substituting it for your other strength workouts once or twice a week, especially if you're feeling any soreness around the knee or ankle joints.

Date	Today's Activity Goal(s)	Total Minutes (or √)	Stretch? (√)	Comments, Other Activities? (vigorous chores, sports, other exercise, etc.)	Estimated Miles Walked
Sunday	cross-train				
Monday	40, strength				
Tuesday	25				
Wednesday	1:00, speed #5				
Thursday	35, strength				
Friday	off				
Saturday	3:00 hike				

Miles this week: _____

Total miles for the year: _____

Make time for your weekend hike

On a weekend when a longer walk or hike is planned, you see that the midweek walks tend to be shorter. This is for two reasons. One is that your body can handle only so much physical stress at a time—it needs opportunities to rest and rebuild around longer and harder efforts.

The second reason acknowledges that you probably have only so many hours in a week to devote to your walking. When a long weekend hike is planned, it can simply make life a bit easier if the rest of the week isn't packed with lots of long efforts.

Tip for the week. **To really ease up the exercise demands on your life this week, sneak in your shorter walks early in the morning or over lunch. Then take advantage of these easier walking days to make sure you're ready to get out and enjoy your hike on Saturday. Have your knapsack, all-weather gear, and other essentials from chapter 9 ready to go (see page 103), and get any maps and food you'll need for the hike.**

	Date	Today's Activity Goal(s)	Total Minutes (or √)	Stretch? (√)	Comments, Other Activities? (vigorous chores, sports, other exercise, etc.)	Estimated Miles Walked
Sunday		cross-train				
Monday		1:00, strength				
Tuesday		35				
Wednesday		1:00, speed #6				
Thursday		45				
Friday		off, strength				
Saturday		1:15				

Miles this week: ―――――

Total miles for the year: ―――――

Maintain your balanced, comprehensive program

You may be having no trouble getting in every workout the program recommends, or you may find it challenging. But whenever you're pressed for time, keep in mind your activity priorities. Make sure to always get in your higher priorities, even at the expense of lower ones when necessary.

Tip for the week. **Here are your priorities, based on the activity pyramid:**
1. **Walk or be active for 30 minutes most days of the week.**
2. **Stretch after your walks as many days as you can.**
3. **Take longer walks (more than 45 minutes) several days a week.**
4. **Add at least two days of strength training.**
5. **Speed up your shorter walks once or twice a week.**
6. **Add variety to your week with cross-training.**

	Date	Today's Activity Goal(s)	Total Minutes (or √)	Stretch? (√)	Comments, Other Activities? (vigorous chores, sports, other exercise, etc.)	Estimated Miles Walked
Sunday		cross-train				
Monday		55, strength				
Tuesday		45				
Wednesday		1:00, 1-mile test				
Thursday		40, strength				
Friday		off				
Saturday		1:30				

Miles this week: _____

Total miles for the year: _____

Check your time for a 1-mile walk again

Head to the track on Wednesday and time yourself for a mile. Warm up with an easy 15 minutes of walking, then blaze through four laps (1 mile) at full speed. Walk easily for the remainder of an hour. Record your time here, then look back at the time you recorded for a mile in week 35. Have you improved? If not, it means either you're already at your maximum fitness (doubtful), you haven't been pushing the Monday and Wednesday speed workouts (well?), or you haven't been paying attention to speedy-walking technique.

Tip for the week. **Here are the four keys to fast-walking technique—you should be using them all the time, but especially during fast efforts:**

1. **Good tall posture and eyes on the horizon.**
2. **Focus on faster steps, and allow your stride length to increase naturally.**
3. **Bend your arms 90 degrees at the elbows; hands trace an arc from waistband to sternum height.**
4. **Push off consciously with your toes at the end of each step.**

	Date	Today's Activity Goal(s)	Total Minutes (or √)	Stretch? (√)	Comments, Other Activities? (vigorous chores, sports, other exercise, etc.)	Estimated Miles Walked
Sunday		cross-train				
Monday		50, strength				
Tuesday		45				
Wednesday		1:00, speed #7				
Thursday		45, strength				
Friday		off				
Saturday		1:15				

Miles this week: ————

Total miles for the year: ————

Let your body (and your training log) be your guide

If you've been tallying your total miles, you've probably noticed that your walking mileage has varied quite a bit from week to week. That's because you're now training at a high enough level that it's beneficial to intersperse easier weeks now and then just to give your system time to recover and rebuild. As you go forward with your walking, listen to your body and follow its advice. If you're feeling sore or fatigued, then maybe you need an easy week. If you're noticing your speed dropping off, it may be time for a few speed workouts. If you find that hills seem to tire you out, it may be time for some leisurely hikes on rolling terrain to build strength.

Tip for the week. **Take advantage of the fact that you keep a training log. Look back and see if there are any lessons to be learned from what you recorded. Look for:**

- **Specific workouts you especially enjoyed (or hated).**
- **Courses or loops that you walked a long time ago. Go back and try them again and see how fast you are now.**
- **Prewalk meals or foods that caused enough trouble that you noted it.**
- **Training weeks that seemed especially hard or easy—what made them feel that way?**

Date	Today's Activity Goal(s)	Total Minutes (or √)	Stretch? (√)	Comments, Other Activities? (vigorous chores, sports, other exercise, etc.)	Estimated Miles Walked
Sunday	cross-train				
Monday	1:00, strength				
Tuesday	30				
Wednesday	50				
Thursday	30, strength				
Friday	off				
Saturday	10K walking event				

Miles this week: _____

Total miles for the year: _____

Do your best in a 10K event

Really try your best in your 10K walk (or whatever distance you've chosen) this weekend—you may be surprised at how many walkers and even runners you beat! One effective strategy is to wait until people are settling into their paces, usually during the second mile, and then pick someone in the distance you're going to work on (that is, try to catch). Choose someone with a brightly colored hat or jersey (it's easier to see) and don't try to catch up all at once—chip away slowly and steadily. It's a great way to push yourself to a fast time, whether you catch your prey or not!

Tip for the week. Compare your pace for the 10K to the pace you held in the 5K walk (week 40). If it wasn't much slower, it's a testament to how much you've improved your strength and endurance over the past eight weeks. If it's faster, then you're a veritable superathlete!

Walking Speed (mph)	Minutes to Walk 1 Mile (min:sec)	Approximate Time for 10K (hr:min:sec)
3.0	20:00	2:04:20
3.5	17:10	1:46:30
4.0	15:00	1:33:10
4.5	13:20	1:22:50
5.0	12:00	1:14:30
5.5	10:55	1:07:50
6.0	10:00	1:02:10

16

The Thrill of Victory: Walking in an Event

You should take part in a formal walking event. This isn't just a recommendation; it's as close to an order as I can give you. It will motivate you as you prepare, you'll have a great time doing it, and in the end you'll enjoy a sense of accomplishment that you richly deserve.

Walkers are finding more formal and informal events open to them every year. Road race directors admit that their running participation is flat, but walking divisions are growing. Charities by the score are holding walks as fund-raisers. And I'm not just talking little 2- and 3-mile fun walks. Ten-kilometer (6.2-mile) events and half marathons are common, and walking full 26.2-mile marathons is all the rage. Walking events are hot, and with good reason—they let just about anybody tackle a challenge and feel the thrill of finishing.

You wouldn't necessarily enjoy every type of event that's out there. But you should try one at least once. Here's why you'll like it:

- **Motivation.** Preparing for a walking event gives you a concrete goal and helps keep your training on track.
- **Camaraderie.** Walking in an event exposes you to lots of other walkers. Events are a blast to train for and participate in with someone else. But even if you go it alone, it's likely you'll make new friends along the way.
- **The thrill.** If you've truly given your best effort, I guarantee that you'll be excited and proud at finishing. There's a unique, tremendously satisfying thrill to crossing a finish line and knowing you've done it yourself. It's a kind of physical satisfaction that's increasingly scarce in modern life.

Even if you're not Type-A

Not every walking event is a race. In fact, a huge number of events are either fund-raisers or just informal walks. Even running races often have walking divisions that are separate from the run. More important, every event I've ever been to has a wide range of participants. There are competitors up front using racewalking technique (or something like it) to post their best time. But there are also people whose only goal is to finish—and to have fun doing it. In fact, I competed on the U.S. racewalking team, tried out for two Olympic teams, and represented the United States in several lesser international competitions, but I have to admit that one of my most memorable races was one I did purely for fun.

My event was the 50-kilometer (31-mile) racewalk, which you can imagine required a lot of focus and discipline. I enjoyed competition, but races—averaging nearly eight minutes a mile for more than four hours—weren't what you'd call fun. Still, at the end of the competitive season one year about 10 of the country's top walkers and another dozen from overseas were invited to take part in an exhibition competition in the New York City Marathon (a mere jaunt of 26.2 miles). We started 15 minutes before the runners and were asked not to race seriously until at least the 5-mile mark—they wanted us grouped together to increase spectator awareness, apparently. Basically, I took it to mean we were supposed to have fun and please the crowd—and they didn't have to tell me twice.

We were the first to cross the Verrazano Narrows Bridge—a huge thrill with helicopters overhead, fireboats shooting streams of water in the air, and an immense crowd as we came off the bridge into Brooklyn. It was certainly the largest crowd I'd ever racewalked in front of, but it also got me in the mood not to race but to experience the event. I talked to more runners ("Heck, how're you *walkin'* that fast?"), gave more high-fives to kids on the side of the road ("Hey, mister, what you doin'?"), dance-walked past every band (racewalking's especially good for reggae, I found), and perused in great detail one of the world's most amazing cities. When it was all over, I finally understood how the five boroughs fit together and I'd had a complete blast—and I still did a respectable time (about 3 hours and 50 minutes, faster than two-thirds of the runners).

Maybe you won't walk the New York City Marathon—and maybe you will—but I hope that you'll walk in at least one event to experience some of the fun that you won't get out in your workouts alone. Of course, not everyone would enjoy the structure and utter tumult of a big-city marathon. So here's a quick sampling of some events out there that you might like to try, listed from least to most structured. For contact information and details, see the resource list at the back of this book under "Events."

Volksmarches

- **What are they?** Usually 10K (6.2-mile) noncompetitive walks on trails and through communities, often in scenic or historic areas. Occasionally shorter (5K) and longer (up to 50K) distances are offered.

- **Who hosts?** Events are organized by local chapters of the American Volkssport Association (AVA), a national member-based walking organization.

You Might Like	You Might Not
Relaxed, family-oriented environment.	Very low key—sometimes you'll feel like you're barely in a formal event.
Well-organized, well-measured courses.	Great variation in course quality—from very scenic to mundane.
Decidedly noncompetitive if that's what you're looking for.	You're not likely to get pushed to a hard effort or your best time at an AVA walk.

- **Why do it?** To enjoy the outdoors; some people record the number of kilometers they've walked and collect commemorative pins and patches from events.
- **How it starts.** Usually an open start; you can sign up and start at any time during a designated window (for example, 8 A.M. to noon).
- **What it's like.** Very family-oriented, go-as-you-please events. Courses are accurately measured, so some folks walk for speed, but most just enjoy the great settings.

Fund-raising walks

- **What are they?** They range from 1 mile to marathon distance or more; 5K (3.1 miles) is very common. Most fund-raisers focus on a noncompetitive approach. The goal is raising money and awareness for an important cause.
- **Who hosts?** Groups ranging from local schools and charities to national research organizations, like the American Heart Association.

You Might Like	You Might Not
Wide range of events, causes, and distances to choose from.	You may have to raise a specific (even substantial) donation to take part.
Usually well-organized events, often with entertainment or other activities.	Some variation in course accuracy; can't always be certain of your time.
Often have a range of competitive attitudes, so you may find folks at your level.	Some folks find the cause-related element overly pervasive.

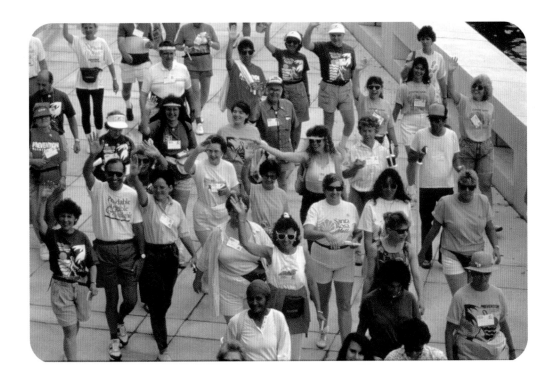

- **Why do it?** Many fund-raiser participants have a close personal association with the cause—knowing someone affected by the disease, or a child attending the beneficiary school, for example.
- **How it starts.** Often these events request that you arrive for a mass start (everyone at once), but this varies.
- **What it's like.** Most are loose and inviting, and competition is downplayed; many disease-related fund-raisers are quite emotionally charged around the cause.

Running races

- **What are they?** Races on roads or trails over practically every distance from 1 mile to 100; 10K (6.2 miles) is very common now.
- **Who hosts?** Some are for charities, but many are organized by local running clubs that use the events for fun, competition, and to build awareness; some partner with walking clubs to put on the walking portion.
- **Why do it?** Competition is the primary goal—seeing how fast you can cover the distance.
- **How it starts.** All at once with the firing of a gun or shout of "go." Sometimes the walkers start separately—five minutes before or after the runners, for example. But other races simply require that walkers start at the back of the running pack—no bargain if you're looking for an accurate time for your effort, because it may take minutes after the clock is started to actually reach the starting line (Have your watch ready to time yourself).
- **What it's like.** Races vary widely, so ask questions before signing up. Is there a separate start for walkers? Do walkers get the same T-shirts and refreshments as runners? Are walkers' results and times segregated from the runners'? Are walkers in the random prize drawings? If you'll be treated as a second-class citizen, don't bother walking in the event.

You Might Like	You Might Not
Often the most charged, exciting settings, with spectators and competitors to push you if you want to go fast.	Walkers can be an afterthought in organization and prizes.
Well-organized, well-measured (often certified) courses.	Can get trampled by runners, depending on the start and design of the course.
There's nothing better than beating a runner—while you're walking!	Some runners are downright indignant when they get passed by a walker.

Racewalking events

- **What are they?** Races usually at 5K, 10K, and 20K distances, as well as the occasional 50K or odd mileage distance.
- **Who hosts?** Usually local racewalking clubs, or regional chapters of the national governing body for racewalking, USA Track and Field.

- **Why do it?** Competition and camaraderie. Racewalkers are a fraternal bunch, and they see races as both athletic and social gatherings.
- **How it starts.** Like other races, with the firing of a gun or shout of "go."
- **What it's like.** Judges actually watch to see that you maintain legal technique (see chapter 17), but most local events welcome newcomers with open arms, and offer instruction rather than disqualification if you haven't mastered the technique.

You Might Like	You Might Not
Generally well-organized, warm, and inviting events.	They can be extremely low key, with just a handful of competitors and supporters.
A great chance to learn about racewalking and boost the intensity of your workout.	A very specific and somewhat technical event, which requires some work to master.
Adds a technical element, and truly turns walking into a competitive sport.	You never know if there will be one wacko yelling at the judges that his technique is fine!

Multiday events

- **What are they?** A fairly new phenomenon on the walking circuit, multiday walks often require walking from 10 to 40 kilometers (6 to 25 miles) several days in a row.
- **Who hosts?** Groups have sponsored multiday events as fund-raisers (for example, the Avon 3-Day Breast Cancer Walks), but this is also a format used by the International Marching League (IML), an international organization like the AVA that hosts noncompetitive, multiday walks in magnificent locations around the world (see "Events" in the resource list).
- **Why do it?** Many IML participants are gathering international patches and commemorative stamps along with having lots of fun. Fund-raising events for diseases seem to focus on commemorating the struggles of those facing the affliction and raising awareness.

You Might Like	You Might Not
A physical accomplishment that you'll be proud of for a lifetime if you finish.	Muscle soreness, blisters, chafing, calluses, dehydration, exhaustion—these events are hard!
Usually highly organized operations, often with support for moving your gear, meals, accommodations, etc.	Requires lots of logistical preparation— don't sign up on a whim.
Guaranteed to get you in great shape and help you walk off some pounds.	To do it right, you should invest a lot of training up front so that lack of fitness doesn't limit your chances.

- **How it starts.** These events generally give you the flexibility to get going when you want, as long as you'll finish by a designated time each day.
- **What it's like.** The ups and downs of a shared struggle. Over several days there is time for lows as you suffer blisters and fatigue, but also the highs of new friendships and a huge sense of accomplishment.

Walking in Your First Event

Walking in your first event will be fun no matter what. But you can impress your friends and fellow walkers and seem like a seasoned pro if you follow this checklist. You'll also be more likely to have a successful walk, free of injuries or unpleasant surprises. These tips are targeted for longer, more structured events such as a 10K road race or even a marathon, but the checklist can guide your planning for anything from a 5K on up. Of course, for shorter walks you don't need quite as much training time up front; nor do you need to think as much about details like eating extra carbohydrates before or during the walk. But for any walk of more than two hours, follow the nutritional tips; if it'll be more than four hours, start your training a month or two earlier.

First

- **Pick out your event.** Learn as much as you can up front—what time of day it is, whether the course is hilly or flat, whether you start and finish in the same place, and if water or other aids will be provided along the course.
- **Tell people you're doing it.** Making a public vow commits you to the event, and to training for it; you may even find a walking partner.

Three Months Before

- **Get an entry form and sign up.** Actually paying your entry fee locks it in and should help you stick with your preparations even more.
- **Plan your training.** Use a program like the one outlined at the end of this section of the book. If it's a marathon, start a month earlier and use the training program at the end of chapter 19.
- **Get a calendar, mark the date, and count backward.** Actually write in your most important workouts each week. Note the longest and the two fastest walks you'll try to do each week, then use the calendar as a log, marking each workout as you complete it.
- **Recruit a training partner.** Now is the time to find a friend, family member, or coworker to walk with you. Once you get a yes, fill out an entry form and send it in—then your partner is hooked, too.

Two Months Before

- **Strengthen your walking-specific muscles.** Sometimes your smallest muscles cause the biggest problems when you tackle your first long event. Your big muscles get trained by your daily walks, but small muscles of the feet, ankles, and hips remain susceptible to collapse. So include the ankle and knee exercises in chapter 10 twice a week, or the full preventive exercise routine in chapter 18.
- **Buy and break in your shoes.** Don't wait until the last minute to decide which shoes you'll wear. Buy a new pair well before event day and use them once or twice a week. Start with shorter walks, then use them in your longest workouts to make sure you're comfortable and blister-free.
- **Try lots of different pre-event meals.** Even if it's a morning event, you'll want to put some food in your stomach before your walk. On your long weekend walks try lots of different things—bananas, bagels, toast, tea—and see what works well in your stomach and leaves you feeling energized.

The Month Before

- **Try out your clothes.** Be sure you've worn everything you intend to use in the race and have checked for tight spots and chafing seams.
- **Go check out the course.** If you're not familiar with where your walk will be and it's a short enough drive, go visit the course. Ideally, you can even do one of your last long weekend workouts on a portion of the course.

The Week Before

- **Cut back your workouts.** Elite athletes call it tapering—in the final 7 to 10 days before the event shorten your training walks (by 30 to 50 percent) while maintaining your speed. You'll rest your body but remain sharp.

Two Days Before

- **Start nibbling carbohydrate snacks.** For any event more than two hours long, do some snacking beyond your normal healthy meals throughout the day.

- **Start drinking plenty of water.** All day you should be sipping water so your body is well hydrated before you even start the race.

The Day Before

- **Pick up your race participant's packet and number.** Take note of special instructions, course changes, and how water and aid will be administered.
- **Know how you're getting to the start on race morning,** where you need to be, and when. Double-check.
- **Know what you're going to do with your warm-up gear.** If you wear sweats to the start, know where you'll put them (in your car, at a race baggage check).
- **Pack a race morning packet.** Include a small container of petroleum jelly for toes and chafing; a water bottle to keep sipping; extra safety pins; sunglasses, hat, and sunscreen; toilet paper; and a last snack (say, a bite of bagel) just in case.

The Night Before

- **Pin your number to your jersey.** Lay out the clothes you'll wear. Then relax and enjoy dinner; go to bed at a reasonable hour, but not insanely early.
- **Don't underestimate the weather.** If it's hot, plan for it with sunscreen, a hat, and lots of water. But if cold or rain looms, bring a hat and gloves and wear a long-sleeved shirt or tights. Once you're well into the race, a small drop in temperature or a bracing wind can really sap your energy. It's easy to take off layers you don't need, but you can't put on what you don't have.

Race Morning

- **Eat breakfast.** Food you're familiar with and have tested on the mornings of long workouts.
- **Get to the start a little early.** Don't get there so close to the start time that you feel rushed or don't have time to loosen up a little—but don't worry about a long warm-up.

Race Time

- **Don't start too fast.** It's the fatal flaw, and can happen if you get sucked along by someone else. Stick with your pace and plans. If you start too slowly and halfway through you feel great, you can always pick up the pace. But start too fast and you may really begin to suffer halfway through.
- **Break the walk into chunks.** Don't think, "Five miles to go." Instead, focus on good walking technique and getting to the next water station or mile marker.
- **Remember to have fun.** Wave to the crowd, talk to fellow walkers. If it's a fund raiser, think about how you're helping others. Enjoy how much you're helping yourself.
- **Be smart.** If despite your timely training and perfect preparations something goes wrong, don't panic, and don't be a hero. If something hurts bad enough to make you walk funny, such as a massive blister or sore hip or ankle, it's probably better to drop out than to try to finish. Being tough and finishing doesn't prove anything, and it can turn a minor irritation into a real injury if you're not careful.

At the End

- **Don't stop immediately.** Walk slowly for a few minutes to cool down, drink some water, and relax with a few minutes of stretching.
- **Stick around for the raffle.** Hey, someone's got to win that dinner for two, right?

If you had told Joanne Dow in 1990 that by the year 2001 she would be have tried out for two Olympic teams, she'd have asked when your next flight to Mars was. A capable collegiate swimmer, Joanne figured her jock days were over when she graduated. After getting married and having two kids, there was definitely no going back. Or so she thought. As time went on and her kids got older, her part-time work as health club instructor led her to learn more about fitness walking—so much so that she eventually became an instructor.

The Turning Point

In 1993 Joanne showed up at a noncompetitive walking event where she hooked up with members of the New England Walkers, a local racewalking club. Before Joanne knew it, she was competing in local races and doing pretty darn well. After attending a clinic by former national team coach Martin Rudow, she was convinced that even at age 30 she had the key elements for success: fundamentally sound racewalking technique, good athletic talent and fitness, and the willingness to work very hard. Eventually she connected with me for ongoing coaching.

A Week in Her Life

Even though Joanne is committed to minimizing how much disruption her training and competition causes in her family members' lives, she still has to weave in 40 to 60 miles of walking a week, plus daily yoga, two to four weight-lifting workouts, massages, lots of time for preventive icing, cross-training, and travel for workouts and races. After getting her kids off to school, on weekday mornings she tends to do her easier workouts (usually 5- to 8-mile walks) and cross-training. Her weekly long workout (12 to 15 miles plus requisite stretching and icing afterward) typically blows half of Saturday. Another day of the week is wiped out by a trip to Boston for a killer workout on the track. Joanne tackles a third hard weekly workout with a friend who runs with her; and she makes time for swimming and other cross-training.

Her Biggest Accomplishment

It would be easy to say a bronze medal in the 1998 Goodwill Games, fifth place in 1999 Pan Am Games, and being a member of the U.S. World Cup teams in 1997 and 1999. But I'm convinced it's maintaining healthy relationships at home and a balanced perspective on being a top-flight athlete. It's important to try to win, but it's just as important to enjoy the ride.

Her Keys to Success

An extraordinarily supportive husband, and a mind-boggling work ethic.

What's Next?

Spreading the word that if she can find time to devote 30 hours a week to preparing for competition, you can find 30 minutes a day for your health.

17

Racewalking: Your Quickest Route to Fitness

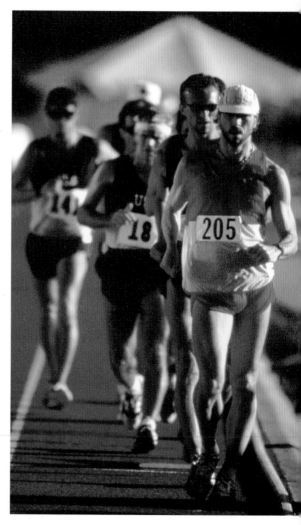

Have you ever seen an overweight racewalker?

How's this for an assertion guaranteed to get an argument: Racewalking may be humanity's best and most natural workout. Wait a minute, you say. You mean that ungainly-looking, high-speed, hip-swinging, arm-pumping walking gait is our best workout? How could that be? Before you pass judgment, hear me out. Here are five reasons racewalking may be your ideal exercise challenge:

1. **Racewalking requires no more gear than a regular walk down the street.** No equipment, no teams, no ice or snow, no courts or playing fields—just a decent pair of shoes and comfortable clothes. To me, that gives racewalking the edge over many equal or lesser cardiovascular pursuits.

2. **Racewalking can be a very vigorous workout.** You can burn as many calories racewalking as you can doing just about any other sport, including fast running. Elite racewalkers tested at the U.S. Olympic Training Center show fitness comparable to elite runners'; the same comparison holds true for recreational athletes in both sports.

3. **The impact and chance of severe injury are fairly low in racewalking.** Even at high speeds, racewalkers hit the ground with only about one and a half times their body weight—most runners pound the earth with three or four times their body weight. Acute injuries ap-

pear more likely in running than in racewalking at fitness-inducing speeds. Why? See the next reason.

4. **It's actually—get ready for this—a fairly *natural* movement.** Racewalking is just an extension of the things humans naturally do to walk faster, taken to their highest level. Make someone walk fast on a treadmill without instruction and she'll take faster steps, bend her arms, and extend her stride. Racewalkers do all of this, but make it a smoother, more rolling gait for greater efficiency. And no, it doesn't hurt your knees (because the loads are low) or hips (which are ball-and-socket joints with plenty of range for the movement).

5. **The rules are actually perfectly logical.** Okay, this is where I may lose you, but keep this in mind—all sports have rules, and some of them are pretty arbitrary. Why, exactly, is it three strikes in baseball and four downs in football? Why do high jumpers have to take off from one foot? (Yes, they do.) And could anybody in the world explain how they do that scoring in gymnastics and figure skating? In racewalking the rules actually reflect the fundamental difference between a walk and a run. The rest of the movement is based on efficiency, nothing more.

Two rules to walk

There are two rules for competitive racewalking, which have evolved over at least 200 years. We know this because there are records of formal walking races dating to the late 1700s. In fact, early walking races were long-distance affairs (and the focus of much wagering), with full reporting in the newspapers; the sport's stars were household names. Some of the early feats were astonishing—such as that of Captain Robert Barclay, who walked 1,000 miles in 1,000 consecutive hours in 1809. Obviously, at such distances breaking into a run wasn't an issue—keeling over exhausted was. In the 1906 Olympics racewalks were included at sprint distances of 1,500 and 3,500 meters (about 1 and 2 miles), necessitating clearly stated rules so that judges could disqualify athletes who broke from a walk to a run. These rules have evolved, as have the Olympic distances, which now stand at 20 kilometers (12.4 miles) for women and men, and 50 kilometers (31 miles) for men.

Rule 1. One foot must always be in contact with the ground. That means the heel of your front foot has to touch the ground before the toes of your back foot come off.

This rule is pretty intuitive, and it reflects what you'd notice if you could watch yourself walking (normally) and running down the street. When you run, you're actually airborne during every stride, literally jumping from one foot to the other. When you walk you never actually leave the ground; one foot or the other (and, briefly, both) is always touching. It's the first and most obvious difference between a walk and a run.

Rule 2. The knee of your supporting leg must be straight from the moment your heel strikes the ground until it passes vertically under your body.

That means the leg you're standing on has to be straight from the instant it touches the ground until it's straight up and down underneath you; then it can bend. This makes your leg slightly longer than in normal walking, in which your leg bends a bit as you stand on it. It explains some of the hip action in walking—your hips roll to accommodate a slightly "longer" (actually straighter) leg than usual. But why have a straight-leg rule at all?

Think again of running versus walking. In running you jump from step to step. In fact, you're bouncing, because each time your leg hits the ground it bends at the ankle, hip, and (especially) knee to absorb the energy of impact. Some of this energy gets stored as your tendons and muscles stretch like rubber bands, and then gets used as you bound into the next step. Your leg acts a little like a spring, absorbing energy as you hit the ground and giving it back as you bounce up for your next stride. The bending of your knee is critical to this rebound action.

Meanwhile, in a normal walk practically no spring action occurs in the leg. You simply fall from one leg to the other in a very smooth way, with much less bending and springing of the knees. The rules of racewalking simply reflect this difference by mandating that your supporting leg—the one touching the ground—be straight as you stand on it. That assures the second big difference between a walk and a run is maintained—it makes sure your legs can't act as springs.

It's easier than you think— and worth the effort

Why even bother to master racewalking, especially if you're already a capable fast walker? Because no matter how good you are, you're going to hit your speed limit. That's a biomechanical fact, and the walking speed limit for regular walking is about 4.5 miles per hour. Add elements like bent arms, very quick steps, and a slightly exaggerated stride and you may stretch it to 5.5 miles per hour for short distances. But to do a full workout at these speeds, you need the real thing—racewalking.

The advantage is that you then open the door to walking as fast as your fitness will carry you. Aerobic fitness and calorie burning galore are there for the taking once you've broken the 5-mile-per-hour speed limit. Of course, initially you may not be fit enough to maintain such high speeds for very long, but with racewalking you'll have the technique to carry you to 10 minutes per mile and faster. That's means burning 800 calories per hour and more, and a vigorous total-body workout, too.

You already know how to racewalk

Think back to the image of young children running around a pool and being told by a lifeguard to walk, not run. Imagine their upright posture, quick steps, fairly straight legs, and bent arms. No one told them the rules of racewalking. But there they are, walking fast but bumping into the speed limit because they haven't learned the finer points of racewalking.

Rather than argue that they should be more like racewalkers, I'm arguing that you should be more like them if you want to racewalk. Turn off your brain and don't try too hard; just try this simple three-step process. Start by getting a visual image of racewalking in your mind. At least think of the kids at poolside, but ideally have a look at a video or photo sequence of the racewalking stride. Better yet, go to an event and see some racewalkers.

1. After warming up during one of your walks, start jogging at a pace just faster than your fastest walking pace. Do this for 20 or 30 strides, then . . .
2. Break into a racewalk and *maintain your speed.* Don't think about technique tips or arm action or anything. Just try to keep moving at the same speed as you were jogging, but break into a walk while doing it.
3. Keep it up for 50 to 60 yards, then go back to a quick jog for a while. Think again about fast walking, hear the imaginary lifeguard's whistle, and break into a walk again.

Repeat this cycle several times.

Walk Talk: How do I pick a qualified walking instructor or coach?

This is a tough question, because there are lots of different kinds of experts out there, depending on what you're looking for. But here are three different types of help you might find, based on your experience and goals:

1. General fitness instruction.
Levels: Beginner to intermediate exercisers.

If you're relatively new to exercise, or are looking for fairly broad instruction, you should seek out a certified fitness instructor or personal trainer who can help with motivation and getting started, assessing your initial fitness, planning an exercise program including walking, stretching, weight training, and instruction in doing things properly. Several organizations offer certifications in the field, including the American Council on Exercise (ACE), Aerobic Fitness Association of America (AFAA), IDEA, and the American College of Sports Medicine (ACSM, which is probably the most rigorous). Ask if your instructor has a master's degree in exercise science—which suggests a more complete background—and ask for references so that you can speak to other clients or students.

2. Walking workout guidance and technique instruction.
Levels: Intermediate to advanced fitness walkers.

More than general fitness instruction, you want someone who has experience working specifically with walkers. There are no formal certifications in walking instruction from the major fitness organizations, but Reebok created a walking instructor program (WalkReebok) that's offered at many health clubs, YMCAs, and YWCAs across the country. The instructors are generally certified fitness instructors who have then taken further training and can therefore be helpful in teaching you how to improve your fitness-walking technique and planning more challenging workouts. Some, but certainly not all, have some formal racewalking experience.

3. Racewalking instruction and coaching.
Level: Advanced fitness walkers or anyone looking to learn racewalking technique.

Formal certifications are less important than availability, experience, and references at this level. There are still relatively few highly qualified racewalking coaches in the United States, but you're most likely to find them affiliated with a local or regional walking or track club (see "Racewalking" in the resource list at the end of this book). Don't assume that just because someone was a good racewalker, he'll make a good instructor. Ask other people who've attended the coach's clinics or training sessions to see if they've found them valuable. Good coaches won't be self-taught—they'll have formal training in exercise science or physical education, perhaps general experience coaching track and field, and at least some personal experience as a competitor (perhaps as a racewalker, but not necessarily). Attend a group clinic or seminar to see the instructor in action before spending money on individual coaching sessions.

Often people who are learning how to racewalk begin by walking slowly, then trying to go faster and faster until they feel they'll break into a run. But my approach is the exact opposite. Instead, I want you to get up to full speed by running, then break into a walk. Amazingly, it seems to work for lots of folks I've coached. It's not going to teach you the finer points of racewalking; in the end, these will come only from working with a coach or other walkers. But to get the hang of the basic racewalking technique, this run-to-walk transition seems to work as well as anything.

It's not a shimmy, it's drive

Though the best way to master racewalking technique is to work with other walkers and get real-life instruction, it's worth knowing in advance the elements of good racewalking technique. All of the things you've learned about fast walking still hold true—they're just taken to a higher, faster level with these additional tips, from top to bottom.

- **Compact, quick, and powerful arms.** The arm swing in racewalking is critical to faster steps, so it has to be a focused and forceful action for greatest benefit. Don't let your hands rise above chest height in the front, and drive your elbows back, not upward, on the back-swing. Your thumb should still rub your waistband as your hand swings back, too.

- **Feel the tow rope.** An image that works for many people is the feeling that a tow rope (like in waterskiing) is attached to their navel and pulling them forward. This gives you the sense of a very slight forward lean—but it's more allowing yourself to fall forward into each step than an actual forward lean. This helps keep your effort directed forward, not up and down.

- **Drive the hips front to back, not side to side.** Caricatures of racewalkers show lots of side-to-side sashay. But watch a world-class athlete and you'll see that the hips are mostly driving front to back, not sideways. This serves to lengthen your stride without making you reach forward with your heel. Just rotate the hip forward a bit on each step.

- **Roll the hips slightly.** There's also a slight up-and-down (again, not side-to-side) motion of the hips, to accommodate your straight leg as it passes underneath your body. Be careful not to exaggerate this movement—focus more on a smooth forward drive with the hips.

- **Have a "skinny" stride.** The faster you walk, the more one foot tends to land straight in front of the other. This is in part because as your hips rotate to the front, they also swing in toward the midline of your body. This means your legs and feet are closer to landing along an imaginary line directly beneath you.

- **Weight on the balls of your feet.** This goes with the tow-rope image—feeling that your weight is forward on your feet increases the sense of falling into each step rather than reaching forward with your heels.

- **Keep your stride behind you.** Feel as if you're putting your leg down under your body, not out in front. (The more it's in front, the more work you have to do to vault up over your leg.) Your stride will lengthen as you speed up—*do not* try to keep it short. But make the length come from driving your hips forward and back, and extending your ankle and pushing vigorously off your toes at the end of each step.

- **Fast steps are the way.** World-class athletes maintain a pace of 200 steps per minute or faster for entire 12-mile races. To really racewalk, you're going to want to reach at least 150 steps per minute. Consider it the minimum necessary to break the 5-mile-per-hour speed limit.

Your best bet for an Olympic uniform

There's one more great reason to get into racewalking—so few people do it seriously. Competitions are delightfully relaxed affairs, and newcomers are welcomed with open arms. In fact, don't go to a pure racewalking event unless you're ready for a dozen or so new best friends. The great thing is that most are passionate about their sport and sincerely happy to help someone else learn.

Racewalkers are also generally happy to find potential new training partners. Because the event is both technically and physiologically demanding, you can really benefit from working out with someone else regularly. It gives you a push to walk faster, and it provides someone who can offer observations on your technique.

The sport offers an opportunity to rub elbows and compete with some of the country's best endurance athletes. There are relatively few racewalking events across the country, although regions with active local clubs have plenty of offerings. So when top-flight athletes are looking for training races or hard workouts, they often jump into local competitions—the same 5K, 10K, and 20K races that anyone can sign up for. Only major events like the races at the national track and field championships and selection races for the Olympic team (and other international races) require that you've walked a specific qualifying time.

I think this is one of the joys of truly amateur athletics. Although I suppose it would be great if the top athletes had big corporate sponsorships to support their training—and some people say we'd have a lot better shot at winning Olympic medals with this kind of support—racewalking would lose its egalitarian charm. Since most races are open to all comers, there can be quite a mix of athletes on the course or track during a race—men and women of all ages and abilities. I quite fondly recall the milieu of major championship races in my competitive days. Some of the fiercest contests were often in the senior age brackets (10-year increments over age 40), because the athletes knew each other well and had built long-standing, mostly friendly rivalries. Local recreational athletes often took part and encouraged us even as we lapped them.

Most intriguing is the notion that not only can you rub elbows with nationally competitive athletes, but you might actually become one. In the past 10 years several men and women who came to the sport of racewalking as adults have broken into the top five in the country. Unlike so many sports that require years of experience, often beginning in childhood, racewalking seems well suited to anybody with a decent athletic background who can master the technique. Sure, to be a top competitor demands some fundamental genetic gifts of endurance and strength, and a willingness to work extremely hard. But you'll never know if you have these unless you give it a try.

To prove that this isn't entirely fantasy, consider this: The fourth-place finisher in the 1992 and 1996 Olympic trials 10K racewalk didn't even start racewalking until 1988, in her late 20s. She missed the Olympic team both years by one place (though she did compete on numerous other U.S. teams, including squads racing in the world championships). One of the top-ranked women in 1998 and 1999—a bronze medalist at the 1998 Goodwill Games and fifth-place finisher at the 1999 Pan Am Games—had been a collegiate *swimmer*; she didn't take her first racewalking steps until age 30. So start racewalking today, and maybe that'll be you sneaking into the 2012 Olympic trials.

Walk Talk: I'm having trouble with my racewalk technique. How do I improve?

The jog-to-walk transition may help you get the basics of the racewalking stride, but to master some of the finer points will take some focus.

• **Problem: Stiff hips or a "wide" stride.** If you were racewalking with wet shoes, your footprints should almost fall one in front of the other. If your left and right prints trace two distinct, parallel lines, you have a wide stride; this can be a symptom of stiff hips or an inflexible lower back.

Solution: Walk the line. On top of patient stretching after your workouts, try "walking the line." At a track, walk along one of the lines that mark the lanes. On the straights, consciously try to make each foot land along the line, and actually touch it (just relax on the curves). Concentrate on driving the hips front to back, to help both feet hit the line.

• **Problem: Bent knees.** Some newcomers to racewalking, especially former runners and men over age 40 (and male runners over 40, especially), seem to have trouble getting their legs straight at the knee while racewalking. They may even feel they're pushing the leg into a straight position but be unable to get it all the way there.

Solution: Weight shift exercise. Stand in front of a full-length mirror with your feet touching one another. Straighten your left leg all the way and shift all your weight onto it; leave your right knee slightly bent. Feel your hips shift over your left leg. Now shift your weight onto the right side, locking the right knee and bending the left, and feeling the hips shift right. Begin slowly shifting your weight back and forth as you alternately straighten the supporting leg—look in the mirror to ensure that you're getting the knee straight. Do this for a minute at a time, then two, slowly increasing the speed until you're shifting your weight and straightening your knees just as fast as if you were walking.

• **Problem: Overstriding.** If you're feeling a thud on every step or tightness in your hamstrings (back of the thighs) and lower back, you're probably reaching forward too much on every stride.

Solution: Quick-step drills. Head to a track and do a series of 100-yard (one-straightaway) sprint walks, taking super-fast baby steps. Consciously truncate your stride so it feels unnatural; the goal is to move your feet as quickly as possible and build a habit of fast strides that are long behind you, not in front.

• **Problem: I just can't seem to put it all together.** Even the patented jog-to-walk transition doesn't seem to help you get the basic hang of racewalking.

Solution: Get a coach. It may be that you need a more methodical approach, carefully building the elements of racewalking technique. Check out "Instructors" and "Clubs" in the resources section to find some racewalkers in your area.

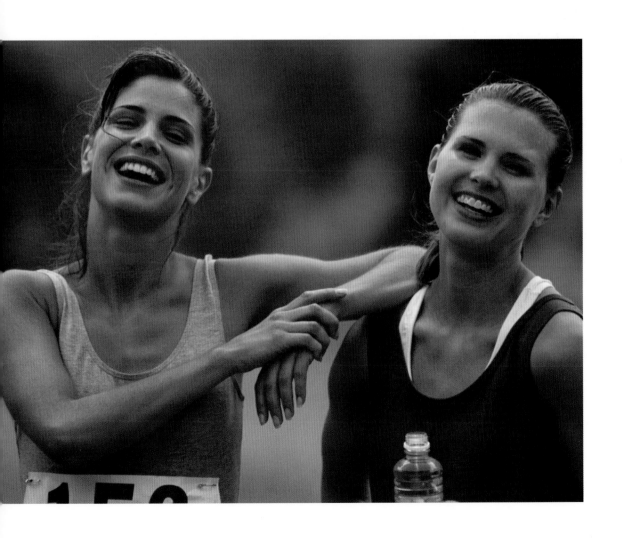

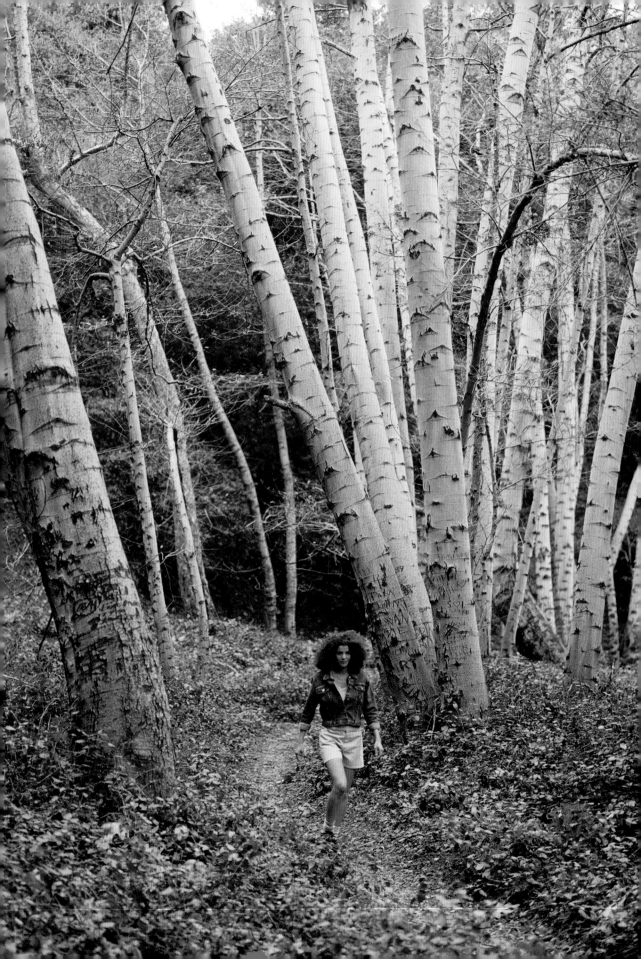

PART IV

Walking for a Lifetime

We can be the transition people, the link between the past and the hope for the future. Our change can affect many, many lives down the road—or I should say, the sidewalk.

RICHARD KILLINGSWORTH
CENTERS FOR DISEASE CONTROL
WALKING MAGAZINE, 1999

18

Keeping an Active Body in Working Order

Avoiding the most common injuries: it starts with prevention

Isn't it ironic that we can take one of our most natural movements—something some people do for an entire lifetime and never give a second thought—turn it into an exercise, and suddenly it becomes rife with physical problems? *Walking injuries*—the phrase doesn't even sound right. Sure, competitive racewalkers training 80 miles a week may get injured. But regular people walking for health and fitness? How can they get injured?

The truth is, they're probably not experiencing actual walking injuries, but either inherent mechanical problems that come to light when the body gets a little more use, or the simple results of doing something irresponsible. Things like trying to walk a lot longer or a lot faster (or both) than the body is ready for, wearing the same pair of shoes for a year and a half, or forgetting to stretch for months on end. So before getting into specific ailments and their solutions, take a look at these dos and don'ts. They may help keep you out of trouble in the first place.

Dos

- Build adequate muscle strength. First and most important is abdominal and torso strength, to protect the back. Muscles around the hip, knee, and ankle joints are the next priority.
- Warm up. Start physical activity gradually, and build intensity only once your body is ready for it.
- Stretch adequately and regularly. Always be well warmed up before stretching.
- Maintain a healthy body weight. Excess weight is tough on the legs, especially the knees.
- Use a knapsack to carry things when walking. Wear both shoulder straps for better back health.
- When doing squats, lunges, or leg presses, avoid locking your knees completely. Use low weight and high repetitions.
- Replace your shoes often—at least every three to five months or 300 to 500 miles, whichever comes first (err low if you're heavy or tough on shoes).
- Back off from activities such as walking hills or knee-bending exercises if they cause you pain.

- Always see a doctor if you experience pain that's not relieved by several days of rest, ice, massage, and elevation.

- Wear shoes appropriate for the activity: walking shoes for walking, basketball shoes for basketball. Seek good medial (inner-heel) support if you overpronate (your feet roll in excessively); look for lots of cushioning if you underpronate.

- Cross-train. Do two or three activities on a regular basis to balance out the body.

Don'ts

- Don't ignore or exercise through pain.

- Never overdo unfamiliar activities.

- Don't exaggerate your stride, overarch your back, or lean forward excessively.

- Don't carry heavy loads in a pack slung over one shoulder, carried in one arm, or balanced on one hip—it's tough on the spine.

- Don't lock your knees while you're exercising on an elliptical trainer, exercise bike, stair climber, or similar devices; be especially careful if you're pregnant, because hormonal changes allow for more lax ligaments around the joints.

- Never give up on exercise completely because of pain; first check with your doctor about alternative activities.

- Don't forget that overall stability, torso strength, and proper posture are key to joint health.

Taking care of the big three: shins, knees, and back

Three areas seem to be the most common trouble spots for walkers.

1. **Shins.** Shins are a common hot zone, especially for beginning fitness walkers or those really trying to ramp up their speed. The muscle on the front of your shin (tibialis anterior) doesn't get a lot of exercise in regular daily life. But in speedy walking it has to do the work of lifting the toes on every step and gradually lowering your foot to the ground as it smoothly rolls from heel to toe with each step. The typical complaint is a tight or burning sensation that comes on fairly early in a walk, but this eventually eases somewhat. The remedies are straightforward and usually quite effective.

   Warm up: Remember to do prewalk warm-ups. Ankle circles (chapter 1) are ideal.

   Stretch: After the shins are warm, stretch them and the calves gently and gradually.

   Strengthen: Increase the strength of these underdeveloped muscles with up-side-back-downs (below) and footsies (chapter 9).

   Go easy: Ease up on your mileage and speed until the strength work kicks in (after a couple of weeks).

   Up-side-back-downs: Move through these four positions 5 to 10 times, holding each position for a 2-count. Do these standing with your feet hip-width apart. These positions strengthen and stretch both the front and the back of the shin, which will help a great deal.

   - Up—stand up on your tiptoes.
   - Side—roll your feet onto their outside edges.
   - Back—lift your toes as high as you can and stand on your heels.
   - Down—stand normally with feet flat, to rest.

2. **Knees.** The knee is a complex joint, and so are most of its problems. There's no simple answer to avoiding knee pain, but the dos and don'ts above get at the most common causes of problems. I'm a strong believer that straight-knee leg lifts (shown in the following strength routine) are one of the best preventive exercises for knee health, and all six of those moves are very well suited to maintaining healthy, pain-free knees. Also, be sure that you're wearing high-quality shoes and getting new ones regularly. The knee is one of the first parts of the body to complain when shoes are overworn.

3. **Back and hamstrings.** These are grouped together only because tightness in the lower back can lead to tightness in the hamstrings (the back of the thighs) and vice versa. My experience suggests when walkers have problems here, it's due to lack of proper stretching, poor abdominal muscle tone, and poor technique. The technique culprit is often over-striding—reaching for a long stride in front, rather than driving the hip, foot, and toes back to extend the stride behind the body. Stretching and strength issues can be solved with the routine below, combined with the core strengtheners presented in chapter 4.

An ounce (and 15 minutes) of prevention

I've often mentioned that it's important to incorporate variety into your program to keep the stimulus on the body fresh and always eliciting improvements in fitness. This holds true for your strength training as well as your walking. One way to do it would be to intersperse the following six-move injury prevention routine into your strength-training time slot now and then. You might include it in lieu of your strength workout every week or two. You could also actually use this as your strength routine for three or four weeks—ideally along with the three-move core strengthening routine shown in chapter 4—and take a break from your other weight lifting altogether. Then come back to your strength training refreshed from the break and ready for some new exercises.

These six simple exercises target often-neglected areas that support the ankles, knees, and hips, such as hamstrings, quadriceps, lower back, and gluteal muscles. For women in particular, quadriceps muscles may be overdeveloped on the outside compared to the inside, which can pull the kneecap off-balance. To improve this balance and others, do this routine two to three times a week—ideally following a walk, when muscles are warmed up. Finish up with the stretches as part of a cool-down; add the stretch routine from chapter 4, too.

1. **Straight-leg lift.**
   Targets: Quadriceps and hip flexors. Complements the walking motion by working muscles that may be underused, such as the smaller muscles of the thigh and hip.
   Cues: Begin by lying on your back with your right leg straight and extended; the left knee is bent, with the left foot flat on the floor. Contract your right thigh muscles to straighten (but not lock) the knee. Slowly raise your leg until your knees are parallel, then lower it. Repeat 8 to 12 times, working up to 2 sets on each side.
   To advance: Begin holding for a 3- to 5-count in the up position.

2. Wall sit.

Targets: Hamstrings, quadriceps, gluteal muscles, and abdominal muscles. A lower-intensity alternative to squats and lunges.

Cues: Stand with your lower back against an exercise ball about 25 inches in diameter that rests against a wall, or simply with your back against a smooth wall. Your feet are shoulder-width apart and a comfortable distance from the wall. Your body is erect. Slowly bend your knees and lower your body until your thighs are parallel to the floor; keep your knees above (not in front of) your feet, and your stomach muscles contracted to avoid excess sway in the back. Pause at the bottom, then slide back up. Repeat 8 to 12 times, working up to 2 sets.

To advance: Increase the pause at the bottom to 3, 5, or even 10 counts.

3. Bridge.

Targets: Gluteal muscles (buttocks), hamstrings, and trunk, including lower-back and abdominal muscles.

Cues: Lie flat on your back, with your arms by your sides, palms up. Both knees are bent, the feet flat on the floor. Using your abdominal and gluteal (butt) muscles, slowly lift your trunk and hips off the floor with a smooth, controlled motion. Squeeze your buttocks at the top, then slowly lower. Keep pressure on your shoulders, not on your head, and do not push with your hands. If you feel cramping in the hamstrings, you'll know they're working too hard; lower your hips slightly to relieve this tightening. Repeat 8 to 12 times, working up to 2 sets.

To advance: Hold the up position for a 3- to 5-count.

4. Single calf raise.

Targets: Calf muscle for ankle support. Ankle stability is critical to proper knee alignment. This move builds calf strength and ankle stability, as well as body coordination and balance.

Cues: Rest your hand on a chair or against a wall for balance, and lift your left leg into a hamstring curl (shin parallel to the ground); extend your right ankle and lift your body fully up on your toes. Slowly lower and repeat 8 to 12 times.

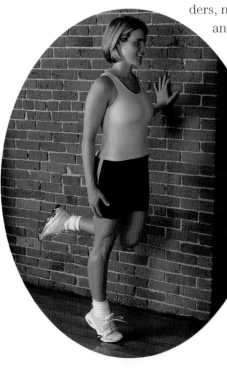

Finishing stretch: After a set, step forward with your right leg, keeping your left leg straight and the left heel on the ground, for a gentle calf stretch. Hold for 6 to 8 slow, deep breaths; then repeat the exercise and stretch on the other side. Do 2 sets on each side.

To advance: Add a third set; place your hands on hips to challenge your balance.

5. Quadriceps stretch.

Targets: Quadriceps, hip flexors (front of the thigh and hip), and shin.

Cues: Lying on your side, with your hips and shoulders stacked, pull the toes of your top foot toward the buttocks with the top hand. If you have trouble, use a towel or T-shirt to extend your grip. Your foot doesn't have to reach your buttocks; pull to the point of feeling a gentle stretch, not pain. Keep your knees in alignment, then slowly pull the top knee slightly behind the other knee, while maintaining stacked hips. Hold for 6 to 8 slow, deep breaths. Repeat 2 to 3 times on each side.

6. Modified hurdler's stretch.

Targets: Hamstrings, gluteal muscles, lower back.

Cues: While seated, extend one leg straight (do not lock the knee) and place the bottom of your other foot against that knee. Holding your shoulders and hips square and your back straight, slowly lower your torso toward the straight leg. Do not collapse through your chest or round your back. Gentle pressure on the bent leg will stretch the inner thigh. Hold for 6 to 8 slow, deep breaths; repeat 2 to 3 times on each side.

But what if you do get hurt?

The fact is, no amount of prevention in the world can ensure that you won't get hurt. Even if you do nothing wrong—you wear the right shoes, stretch and strengthen adequately, increase your mileage gradually—you can still step on a rock funny while hiking and twist your ankle. This is a natural and reasonable risk of active living. So what should you do when an injury occurs?

Ice works wonders

I first realized that even walking wasn't without its aches and pains during my days as an athlete. From the mild soreness that followed a day of climbing to tendinitis or the inflammation of a twisted ankle, ice was—and still is—the treatment of choice. Not only can it give quick pain relief but, applied regularly, the cold will also reduce inflammation and thus allow quicker healing of injured tissue. In my competitive days a common practice was to hold ice in a towel or plastic bag or rub water frozen in a Dixie cup right on the injury. Even more clever, we thought, was a bag of frozen peas, which eventually took on the shape of the injured area.

Enter the 21st century. I now coach an athlete who, when recovering from knee surgery, was walking around with a space-age Aircast Cryo/Cuff. Don't let the name deceive you; ice and cold water still do the work of reducing inflammation. But this device gently compresses the injured area within a flexible fluid-filled sleeve. She could replenish the cold water at will through tubes hooked to a detachable cooler, and 20-minute bouts of icing spread frequently throughout day—the common recommendation—kept her postsurgical inflammation to a minimum.

Even if you're not in surgical recovery, a modern cold pack for the freezer is a good idea for workout soreness and preventive icing. Look for one that's soft, flexible, wraps around the area, and has straps to hold it in place. A material such as polyurethane won't sweat as much when the ice melts, and gel has an advantage over water in that it's flexible right out of the freezer. It may even be better than peas. (For manufacturers, see "Ice" in the resource list at the end of this book.)

An example of the full treatment: plantar fasciitis

Is ice alone enough to treat an injury? Probably not—in fact, most injuries respond best to a full course of conservative treatment. A good example is plantar fasciitis, a chronic condition that can plague people for months or even longer. I'll use it as an example since it's so common.

I can confirm from frustrating personal experience that plantar fasciitis—inflammation and tightening of the sinewy tissue (plantar fascia) that runs along the bottom of your foot—takes real discipline to cure. It can be painful and frustrating, and it's characterized by especially severe tightness first thing in the morning, after your feet have been inactive. Untreated plantar fasciitis can even lead to heel spurs, a hardening of the irritated tissue beneath the heel. The key is sticking with all the elements of treatment simultaneously and patiently curtailing your walking until you're completely clear of symptoms. A sports medicine podiatrist or physician (it's worth seeing one) is likely to suggest all of these:

• **Rest.** Back off on your exercise walking and stay away from high heels, uncomfortable dress shoes, or anything that aggravates the injury until the pain subsides entirely.

• **Ice.** Massage directly on the injured area, 10 minutes on, 20 minutes off, several times a day. End with a warm washcloth to loosen up before walking around. (See "Ice" in the resource list.)

• **Anti-inflammatories** such as aspirin, ibuprofen, and naproxyn sodium. Follow directions carefully, and be sure to take them with food to avoid stomach irritation. (Note that acetaminophen, found in Tylenol, is not an anti-inflammatory, so it's not helpful in this role.)

• **Gentle stretching** of the foot and calf. Stretch only when you're warmed up, after moderate activity such as easy walking.

• **Heel inserts,** normally only 0.25 inch thick or so, cushion and lift the heel slightly and reduce strain on the inflamed tissue.

• **Walking shoes** should be new, well cushioned, and supportive; they should flex only in the forefoot, where the foot bends, and not at all through the arch.

Keep this final point in mind when treating any injury: Be patient. Several weeks of treatment and rest may seem interminable, but it's a lot better than months of nagging pain and missed walks. Staying active can help. It will keep you fit and even hasten healing by helping maintain blood flow to the injured area. Just pick activities that avoid stressing the injury. Low-impact choices such as swimming, yoga, and upper-body weight lifting often fit the bill.

	Date	Today's Activity Goal(s)	Total Minutes (or √)	Stretch? (√)	Comments, Other Activities? (vigorous chores, sports, other exercise, etc.)	Estimated Miles Walked
Sunday		20				
Monday		40, core+				
Tuesday		30				
Wednesday		40				
Thursday		20, core+				
Friday		off				
Saturday		1:00				

Miles this week: ⎯⎯⎯⎯⎯

Total miles for the year: ⎯⎯⎯⎯⎯

A week of healthy walking

Sometimes you have to head back to basics. This will seem like an easy week—but recall that it's the "pinnacle" you were building up to during the first weeks of the program, as you tried to build a healthy walking habit. Now no doubt you'll instinctively cover the 20- and 30-minute walks at a brisk pace, and you may even find yourself chomping at the bit to go longer on the weekend.

Tip for the week. Even if you've chosen to become a very serious athlete, it's a good idea to return to this level of walking once in a while just for a change. Every three to six months—at the very least once a year—throw in a period of three or four weeks in which you go back to this basic routine. You'll maintain your fitness, but it'll feel like a nice break and keep you eager for more.

	Date	Today's Activity Goal(s)	Total Minutes (or √)	Stretch? (√)	Comments, Other Activities? (vigorous chores, sports, other exercise, etc.)	Estimated Miles Walked
Sunday		35				
Monday		45, strength				
Tuesday		1:00 on trails				
Wednesday		50				
Thursday		35, strength				
Friday		off				
Saturday		Day hike! (2:00+)				

Miles this week: _____

Total miles for the year: _____

A week of hiking and endurance

Sometimes you don't want to have to think about how fast you're going—you just want to enjoy getting there. So this week spend at least two (or more!) of your walks on trails. Don't think about speed; just enjoy the varied terrain and being out walking long enough to actually get somewhere. Use this week anytime you need to prepare for a longer hike. For example, four weeks of this routine would be nice preparation for a backpacking trip.

Tip for the week. **The ideal strength routine to use with this week is the injury prevention program shown in chapter 18 (see page 208). Add the footsies exercise from chapter 9 for additional ankle strength, and it's the perfect complement to spending lots of time on the trail. By the way, take a minute this week to make sure your hiking day pack and 10 essentials (chapter 9) are ready to go for the weekend.**

	Date	Today's Activity Goal(s)	Total Minutes (or √)	Stretch? (√)	Comments, Other Activities? (vigorous chores, sports, other exercise, etc.)	Estimated Miles Walked
Sunday		cross-train				
Monday		50, strength				
Tuesday		45				
Wednesday		1:00, speed #1 to #4				
Thursday		45, strength				
Friday		off				
Saturday		1:15, speed #5 to #8				

Miles this week: _____

Total miles for the year: _____

A week of speed and fitness

This is a standard week to build lots of speed and general athletic fitness. When using this routine, rotate through the speed workouts on Wednesday and Saturday. When speed #4 comes up on Wednesday—the workout that alternates walking intervals and strength moves—skip your strength workout on Thursday. When you do a cross-training activity with lots of strength work on Monday, skip Tuesday's strength work.

Tip for the week. When #8 comes up on Saturday, take the opportunity to try different types of events. One time show up at a noncompetitive AVA walk, another weekend head out to a full-blown racewalking race (see chapter 16 for details on both). Here's a hedonistic tip: Six weeks of this might make a good get-your-body-in-bathing-suit-shape-by-summer program.

	Date	Today's Activity Goal(s)	Total Minutes (or √)	Stretch? (√)	Comments, Other Activities? (vigorous chores, sports, other exercise, etc.)	Estimated Miles Walked
Sunday		cross-train				
Monday		45, core				
Tuesday		30				
Wednesday		alternate activity				
Thursday		30, core				
Friday		off				
Saturday		1:00, speed or trails				

Miles this week: ⎯⎯⎯⎯⎯

Total miles for the year: ⎯⎯⎯⎯⎯

A week of rest and fun

Sprinkle a week like this, or even less, into your program whenever your body or life demands it. What the heck is "alternate activity," you ask? Whatever you'd like it to be—a familiar cross-training activity, or something new, or maybe one of the 10 special suggestions for building a more walkable world found in the final chapter of this book. You decide—you're the athlete now.

Tip for the week. If you've really stuck with this program up to this point, you don't need any more tips. You should feel proud of your accomplishment and confident that you're the capable owner of a healthy, vigorous lifestyle. Now it's up to you to pick. For example, what do you feel like on Saturday? Speed work? A walk on trails? Or something else entirely? Only you can decide—so get out there and have fun!

19

Building Your Own Program

What next?

You've stuck to the program, done every workout, and reaped the rewards. You're leaner, stronger, faster, and more energized than ever. But how will you keep up your success without a day-to-day plan for next year? Well, you probably know more about maintaining a program than you even realize. In fact, just a few now-familiar guidelines and tips are all you need to build your own daily walking schedule. But it's really a five-step process—and you can reapply it every two months to help you create your own ongoing plan.

Step 1. Buy a calendar or logbook

Make sure it has plenty of room for writing down your daily program. Or simply draw a sample month and make copies—you could keep them in a folder or binder.

Step 2. Pick a goal

It's easiest to do this if you know what you want to get out of your walking. This year you've followed a program designed first to build overall health, then to help you reduce to a healthy weight or maintain one if you're already there, and finally to build athletic fitness. However, even though these are admirable goals, they may not be what you want for next year or even the next two months. For example, if you're more pressed for time, you may be willing to settle for a basic stress reduction and health maintenance program. On the other hand, if you've been truly inspired you may want to tackle a more aggressive athletic conditioning plan. So consider your goals and available time for the next two months, and pick your targets based on the table on page 218.

You can and should switch your goals from time to time. If you're changing jobs, buying a house, or just plain busy, you may want to focus on level 1, walking for health, for a while. On the other hand, if you have a lot of time and motivation, crank up to the athletic training program, level 3. Just remember to switch to a less intensive program for at least a few weeks every 8 to 10 months to give your body a chance to rest.

As well as these general goals—health, weight maintenance, or fitness—it's worth setting more specific goals, as you've seen with this program. Here are some of my favorites, which I've seen work well for others and myself:

Target	Benefits	Average Hours of Walking per Week	*At Least One Day Each Week, Walk	**Over the Week Walk Fast for at Least
1. Stay healthy	Reduced stress and chronic disease risk, and greater energy.	3 to 3.5 hours	45 min.	10 to 30 min. (3.5 to 4.5 mph)
2. Maintain or lose weight	Same as level 1, plus extra calorie burning to help with weight loss and maintenance.	4 to 5 hours	60 min.	35 to 50 min. (4 to 5 mph)
3. Build fitness	Combines levels 1 and 2, plus improved aerobic conditioning and an ever-more-athletic body.	6 hours or more	90 min.	60 min. or more (4.5 mph or more)

* Ideally, this longest walk of the week should be done all at once, not broken up.
** On days when you'll do some fast walking, try to cover at least 10 minutes' worth of your weekly total, even if it's broken into one- and two-minute bursts.

- Walk 1 mile in 12 minutes. Already got that? Try for 10 minutes, a real challenge!

- Walk a 10K in 75 minutes. That's about 12 minutes per mile, or a 5-mile-per-hour average for a 6.2-mile race. It sounds fast, but it's entirely doable, as long as you work on your speed technique and build the fitness to maintain it.

- Walk a marathon in less than seven hours. If this sounds too easy, make it six hours. Blind-folded. Hopping on one foot. (Okay, I'm kidding about the one foot—you could switch feet.)

- Log 1,000 miles in a year. My mom did this in 1993 and is still proud of the accomplishment. And it's not as daunting as it might seem—it requires an average of about 19 miles a week, or just over 3 miles a day, six days a week. The keys to making it are consistency and good log keeping from the very start. Also helpful, we learned, is a very supportive family come holiday time. When Mom saw the end of year looming and thought she wasn't going to make it, everyone got in on the act of making sure she got her miles in. We either helped her make time or walked with her. In a way, it became a family goal, and we were all very proud when she achieved it. (Well, also sort of relieved. I got my type-A personality from her, and I know it would have been everyone's problem if she hadn't made it!)

- Hike 20 miles in two days. Pick a phenomenal destination, and if you don't feel like backpacking, find a trail with cabins or hostels on the route (see "Hiking" in the resource list at the end of this book).

- Maintain an unbroken streak of some kind of activity every day for six months, or even an entire year. Set a minimum—say, one mile of walking—to count a day.

- Be able to do 25 good push-ups, 10 real pull-ups, or (ideally) both. If these are too easy, up the goals to 50 push-ups and 20 pull-ups.

- Walk the Vierdaagse. That's Dutch for "four days," and it's the granddaddy of noncompetitive walking events. Held each July in Nijmegan, Holland, the four-day march began as a military training exercise in the early 1900s. Now more than 40,000 people (mostly civilians) cover from 30K to 50K each day over the beautiful Dutch countryside—with every village you pass through hosting a full-fledged party! You'll have to train like you've never imagined, but the final walk into Nijmegan on day 4—a combination New York City Marathon finish and miles-long block party with scores of bands and thousands of spectators—makes it all worthwhile. (For more information, log on to www.4daagse.nl.)

Notice that I don't have any weight-loss or fit-into-a-dress sorts of goals. Frankly, these just aren't much fun, and they're not proven to help you stick with it in the long run. Once you get to a size 10, then what? Goals I like focus on the process—it's not the 1,000th mile, it's the 999 you walked all year long to get there! After all, it truly is the route, not the destination, that defines a journey. So pick yourself some exciting routes.

Step 3. Memorize these rules

Do *not* try to write out an entire two-month program. It's time consuming and, unless you're experienced, the weeks will likely get pretty redundant. Instead, just write out what one or two typical weeks might look like, given the weekly totals recommended opposite and your knowledge of your schedule. Follow these rules:

- Walk, or be active in some other way, every day. Remember that even 10 minutes is much better than nothing.
- Alternate easier and harder efforts (shorter days following longer walks).
- Alternate the intensity of your efforts (for example, a moderate pace the day following really fast hills).
- Plan some resistance training at least two days a week. This includes free weights, floor exercises, Nautilus or other resistance machines, or even stretch tubing.
- Try to fit in two, and preferably four, cross-training activities every month.

Step 4. Plan in weekly variety

Times are given in ranges because your program has to be flexible to survive. Some weeks will be better than others; you'll feel better, or have more time on your hands, so shoot for the upper end of the range. When pressed, just be sure to make the minimum goals. This variation from week to week can accommodate a real-world schedule while keeping you from falling into the "if it's Friday, I must be doing 45 minutes" syndrome. Watch out for this kind of repetition from week to week; it can lead to boredom and physical staleness.

Step 5. Get walking, and log it

Now that you've created a "typical" week, start walking and changing it as you go. Remember that you can swap days and workouts to accommodate your schedule. But by keeping a log, you'll be able to monitor whether you still hit your weekly total and get in your key fast walks, long walks, and strength training. Take a look at the final four weeks of the program (weeks 49 to 52). They act as a sample month, cycling through four weekly goals.

It's worth investing in rewards for when you meet your exercise goals—it's proven to increase the chances that you'll keep exercising, and it's just plain fun. Here are a few possible treats—some very affordable, and others a bit extravagant—for you to try:

- **$10.** Plant a fruit tree. Be aware that fruit trees need more attention than even your dog. One pear tree that's about 4 or 5 feet tall costs $8 to $10.
- **$20.** Soak in a hot bath with candles, soothing music, mineral salts, and a glass of decent wine for no less than one hour.
- **$30 to $70.** Attend a sporting event. Watch someone else pant, grunt, and sweat for a change.
- **$35.** Take flying lessons. Some companies offer introductory flights for as little as $35.
- **$70 to $80.** Get a massage. Rub down those tired muscles.
- **$80 to $95.** Rent a limo and have someone else drive you around town. You'll probably even get to play around with the sunroof.
- **$265 to $800.** Stay at a luxury hotel for a night. Check into weekend packages, and don't forget to order room service.
- **$500 to $1,000.** Go to a spa for the weekend. Some offer great package deals during their off-seasons.

Two special programs

Following are two sample programs, designed for very different goals and times in life. The first is an 18-week program designed for someone looking for a serious challenge—walking a marathon. The second is for a woman preparing for one of life's biggest challenges—childbirth. The 18-month program runs from nine months before the baby comes to nine months after, and is drawn from our book, *Walking Through Pregnancy and Beyond*, by Mark and Lisa Fenton (Lyons Press, 2004).

The 18-week marathon training program

If you think you're ready for a marathon but aren't sure you want to obliterate every weekend out walking between now and race day, have I got the program for you! Since walking a marathon at a moderate pace (say, 4 miles per hour) could take up to seven hours, many coaches subscribe to the "time on your feet" training approach. It requires that every weekend you take longer and longer walks, building up to numerous five-, six-, or seven-hour workouts in the weeks leading up to the marathon. Many feel it's the only way to prepare the body for such a long haul. Well, I'm not convinced.

This 18-week program is designed to prepare you to safely and successfully walk a marathon with a relative handful of long weekend training walks. (Before you begin this program, you should be able to complete a sustained 60-minute walk, and several days a week you should be taking 45-minute walks.) The trick is progressively longer workouts on alternate weekends combined with short but challenging fitness-building workouts on weekdays. The midweek workouts boost your maximum speed, which makes walking at a marathon pace feel that much easier, while the weekend efforts are enough to build endurance. Once you've gotten the hang of the midweek speed workouts, you could substitute any of the workouts listed in chapter 14.

But first things first: Once you know the race date, write it down on a calendar. Then begin counting backward, filling in the key workouts from this program for each week. This way you won't be surprised when it's time to plan a long hike in week 13, or a walk of more than four hours in week 15.

The program is built on six days per week of walking: two easy 45-minute walks, plus each of the following key workouts spread over the week. Workouts #1 and #2 are shorter midweek walks, while workout #3 is a longer effort targeted for the weekends; you can swap days to accommodate your schedule as long as you spread the harder efforts out over the week. The program should help most walkers to finish in less than seven hours, and it assumes you don't have limitless hours to train each week. If you'd like to go faster and have more training time, I offer a few tips afterward on how to do so.

Workout #1. Tuesday: Practice speed.

The goal: Improve your ability to maintain target pace.

How: These short but sweet workouts consist of walking as fast as you can maintain for a designated time. Always begin with a 10-minute warm-up and 5-minute cool-down.

Weeks 1 through 5	Start with 10 easy minutes, crank up to a swift pace (an RPE of 7 to 8) for 15 minutes, and finish with 5 minutes to cool down, for a 30-minute total.
Weeks 6 through 11	Increase to 30 minutes of sustained effort after warming up, for a 45-minute total.
Weeks 12 through 16	Bump up to 45 minutes of high speed, and a 60-minute total.
Weeks 17 and 18	Drop back to 30-minute walks with just 15 minutes fast.

Workout #2. Thursday: Build strength

The goal: Increase power in your legs; especially important on a hilly course.

How: During a nonstop 60-minute walk, insert several bursts of either brisk uphill or extremely fast level walking, or both. Begin and end by walking easily for 10 minutes to warm up and cool down. In the first week intersperse just five minutes' worth of intense effort—hard enough to induce heavy breathing—in one- to three-minute chunks. Follow each with a minute or so of moderate walking before the next effort. Add a minute of blistering speed each week: six minutes in week 2, seven minutes in week 3, and so on.

By week 16 your one-hour walk should include 20 minutes of very hard effort sprinkled throughout. Skip this workout entirely in the final week before the race.

Workout #3. Saturday and Sunday: Go long.

The goal: Build endurance, reduce injury risk.

How: Each weekend take progressively longer walks (see the chart on page 222). Occasionally they're broken into two medium-long walks at a quicker pace: one on Saturday afternoon, the other on Sunday morning. The short recovery time enhances the conditioning effect by giving your body less time to repair and reenergize muscles. Be sure to drink water frequently on any effort of more than an hour; nibble snacks on the walks of more than two hours.

Marathon Training Program Log

Columns marked "Easy 1" and "Easy 2" are to check off when you do your two easy 45-minute walks; "Tues." and "Thurs." are to check off when you complete your speed and strength workouts, slated for Tuesday and Thursday, respectively. The times listed assume you're walking in the 4- to 5-mile-per-hour range. If you walk faster than this, then convert these times to mileage using 4.5 miles per hour, and walk the resulting distances for your long workouts.

WEEK	EASY 1	TUES.	EASY 2	THURS.	Saturday Progressively longer endurance walks. (Walk in the P.M. if Sunday walk is an hour or more.)	Sunday Either a 20- to 40-min. recovery walk, or combine with Saturday for more endurance.
1					40 min.	40 min.
2					50 min.	40 min.
3					1 hr.	40 min.
4					1 hr. 15 min.	1 hr.
5					1 hr. 30 min.	20 min.
6					1 hr. 20 min.	1 hr.
7					2 hr.	20 min.
8					1 hr. 30 min.	1 hr.
9					Long hilly hike; at least 3 hr.	20 min.
10					1 hr. 40 min.	1 hr. 20 min.
11					3 hr. 30 min.	20 min.
12					1 hr. 45 min.	1 hr. 15 min.
13					All-day hike: off-road for more than 4 hours	20 min.
14					1 hr.	1 hr.
15					4 hrs. 30 min.	20 min.
16					2 hrs. 45 min.	1 hr.
17					1 hr. 15 min.	40 min.
18					Race weekend!	Walk 26.2 miles

Looking for a Faster Marathon?

You could train for a time of less than six or maybe even five hours by making the following two adjustments to the program:

1. Make it 22 weeks long by repeating weeks 12 through 15, then finishing up with 16 though 18 as shown. The second time through, boost the long Saturday walks in weeks 13 and 15 by a half-hour each.

2. In week 14 (both times you do it) replace the easy Saturday one-hour walk with your best effort in a 5- to 10-mile road race (try for shorter race the first time, a longer one the next). Chase some runners! Skip the speed workout the following Tuesday and walk a quick 30 minutes instead.

Eighteen months of walking through pregnancy

Many women have heard that exercise during pregnancy can help them avoid excessive weight gain, especially during the third trimester. Being active can also help speed weight loss after the blessed event. One thing is clear—pregnancy is no reason to stop your walking, and maintaining your weight isn't the only reason. Moderate physical activity may help reduce physical discomfort as you get heavier, help you sleep better, and keep you fit for the physical challenge (there's an understatement!) of delivery. Here are some tips from the American College of Obstetricians and Gynecologists:

- If you're already a walker, don't try to match your regular pace or distance; listen to your body instead.

- Expect a decrease in balance and coordination as your center of mass shifts and ligaments loosen. Pick safer, more level routes, and consider more supportive shoes, because it may be easier to turn an ankle.

- Stay especially cool and well hydrated, because you'll be more likely to overheat. This is important for both you and the baby.

- Most important, be sure to talk to your doctor about your specific needs and program.

    On page 224 is a logical approach to consider:

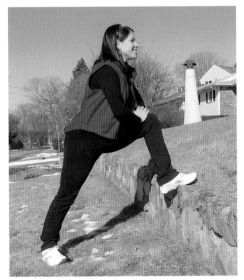

Use warm-ups and a stretch routine to maintain comfort.

		If before pregnancy you		
	Overall	**did nothing, now your average daily goal is:**	**walked 30 mins. daily, now your average daily goal is:**	**walked an hour daily, now your average daily goal is:**
1st trimester	Maintain your program if comfortable.	5 to 15 mins.	Still 30 mins.	Still 60 mins.
2nd trimester	Enjoy the strength you're feeling.	10 to 25 mins.	20 to 30 mins.	40 to 60 mins.
3rd trimester	Break it up over the day if it helps.	10 to 20 mins.	15 to 25 mins.	30 to 45 mins.
0 to 3 months A.B.C.*	Easy first few weeks; then add no more than 5% a week. Try your child in a chest carrier as you feel stronger.	5 to 10 mins.	10 to 20 mins.	20 to 40 mins.
4 to 6 months A.B.C.	Increase 5% to 10% a week; add gentle strength work. Consider an all-terrain stroller for longer walks.	10 to 20 mins.	20 to 30 mins.	30 to 50 mins.
7 to 9 months A.B.C.	Increase 5% to 15% a week; pick up the pace several days a week. Try a baby backpack for trails, once she can hold her head up.	20 to 40 mins.	30 to 40 mins. or more	45 to 70 mins. or more

*A.B.C. stands for "After Baby Comes"

20

The Real Key
to a Life of Health
and Well-Being

Don't walk for exercise

I hope by now you've realized that this isn't really an exercise book. Sure, it's *camouflaged* as an exercise book—walking recommendations, stretches, weight training. But it's really a call for you to change your life. The admonition is simple: Get moving. Don't wait—time is running out on your sedentary life. What should you do? The answer comes in two parts:

1. If you do absolutely nothing right now, start to do *something* regularly—anything physically active—and you'll begin to feel better. If you're already modestly active, then do a little more and you'll feel great.

2. Walking is the activity you should be focusing on. Sure, there are millions of choices, from exercise classes to competitive sports, but for 80 to 90 percent of Americans, they're clearly not working. If you're like most Americans, formal exercise isn't really a dominant part of your life. Walking, however, is. Even if it's just to and from the car, you're *already* a walker. All you have to do is more of it.

So this book is really about making walking part of how you live every day. Not making it exercise. Not a chore. Not a daily obligation. Not even something that takes conscious thought—truly a part of how you live.

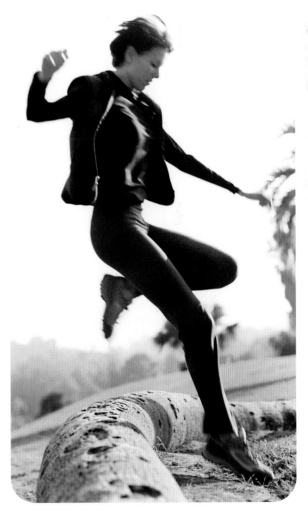

You'll know you've gotten there when a year from now you're doing something downstairs and realize you need something that's upstairs. Maybe you could yell upstairs for your roommate or spouse to throw it down; maybe you could have one of the kids go get it; maybe you could put it off until you went upstairs anyway. But instead you just run up the stairs and get it. Just get up and move without hesitation, without a thought. Because you like moving. Your body feels good moving, and you've simply made moving a part of your life again. When you actually look for chances to move—not ways to avoid it—that's when you'll know you've arrived.

Movement is in your nature— put it in your routine

Here's the big problem with the idea of putting more activity into your daily life: We've spent the last two centuries as a species taking it out. As hunter-gatherers, humans lived an existence that depended on being physically active for survival. If you wanted food, you had to go get it—and that meant working hard. Foraging more than 8 to 10 miles a day or hunting for game is serious work. (Try it sometime—walk 10 miles over broken ground without a trail. In bare feet.) Subsistence-level farming, which is what humans did as they settled into communities, was equally laborious and demanding. Being overweight clearly wasn't the issue—having enough to eat was.

But as we got to be better farmers, and eventually as we entered the industrial age, some societies actually became able to produce more food than they needed. They also began to create time- and labor-saving devices, presumably to improve the quality of life. Everything from automobiles to washers and dryers has given us free time for families, recreation, or more productive work and invention. But in the process these devices have required us to do less and less physical labor.

Forget walking 10 miles a day to forage for food. Now we barely have to walk 10 steps to the refrigerator to make a meal, or (even worse) reach 10 inches to the cell phones in our pockets to order it in. Why make it yourself—let someone else do the work and deliver it, right?

Don't worry, I'm not some Luddite who espouses crushing all of our computers and dishwashers and returning to beating our clothes on rocks to clean them. But I also take very seriously the public health estimates that say we burn 500 to 800 fewer calories a day in routine tasks than we did just 20 years ago. Given that the average woman may burn as few as 2,000 calories a day now (men are closer to 2,700 or so), this reflects a massive change in a very short time.

The answer is clear: We have to find ways to weave activity back into our lives. And it has to be in ways that make activity come as routinely as chasing prey or tilling the soil once did. Walking is the ideal way to do this. In fact, I often use the terms *walking* and *physical activity* or *being active* interchangeably, because walking is already the primary voluntary activity through which most people burn calories on a daily basis.

But routine walking won't happen by accident, and you won't find it easy to do alone. So along with all the motivational tips and ideas threaded through this book about getting yourself to walk and doing it safely and effectively, you have to take one more step. You have to help create a more walkable world. Then walking truly will become a routine part of your life.

Creating a more walkable world

You may think that more sidewalks or trails are the key to a walkable world, and they are. But they're only part of the story. We need places to walk, but if we really want walking to permeate our culture and our lives (and we should), then we need the people around us walking, too. Since it's probably easier to influence the circle of people in your life to begin walking than it is to get sidewalks built, start by looking at the folks you live and work with. If you get them walking, then in the future they can be your allies as you embark on the crusade to get more walking paths and sidewalks and safer streets constructed.

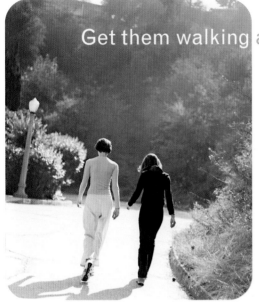

Get them walking at home

There are two critically important reasons to get your closest family and friends walking. One is utterly selfish, the other selfless. If the people around you are walking, they're going to help you build walking into your life. It's a lot nicer and easier to say, "Let's walk downtown to see the movie instead of drive," if you're met by enthusiasm instead of whines. The second reason is that you should care enough about the people around you to want them to feel as good as you do from walking. So how does walking become the household norm? Not by accident; it requires a lot of conscious decisions. Here are some decisions you can make:

• **Never assume you're taking the car.** This may seem utterly simplistic, but it's made all the difference in our household. Whenever we walk out the door to go somewhere, we consciously ask, "How are we getting there?" We first ask if we can walk; if that's not practical, we consider riding bikes. Only if we can't do either do we get in the car.

One of my proudest moments came one drizzly fall morning when my four-year-old son, two-year-old daughter, and I walked out the door to go to our village bagel shop. I opened the car door and my son said, "Awww, no, Dad, let's walk." He far prefers what he perceives as the "normal" way to get downtown: riding his bike and having me push his sister in the all-terrain stroller at a veritable run to keep up (there's nothing like making old Dad sweat—which I did, after we all donned raincoats). His reaction was based on habit—he never assumed we'd ride in the car. Neither should you.

• **Seek out walking destinations.** You're thinking, "That's all well and good for you, Mr. Bagel-Shop-in-Walking-Distance. But I don't have such niceties that I can walk to." Are you sure? Lots of modern American suburbs are largely housing tracts separated from shopping malls separated from industrial parks separated from schools . . . you know the picture. But there are still occasional corner convenience stores, video stores, dry cleaners—lots of places you have to go occasionally. Make these your destinations and go on foot, rather than driving to the giant strip mall. And if the milk costs a little more at the convenience store than at the mega-super-giganta grocery store, so be it—it's still a lot cheaper than what you'd spend on the health club membership that you'd never use anyway. Think of walking trips to the corner video store as your new membership—your membership in your community. (Think of saved gas and wear and tear on the car, too.)

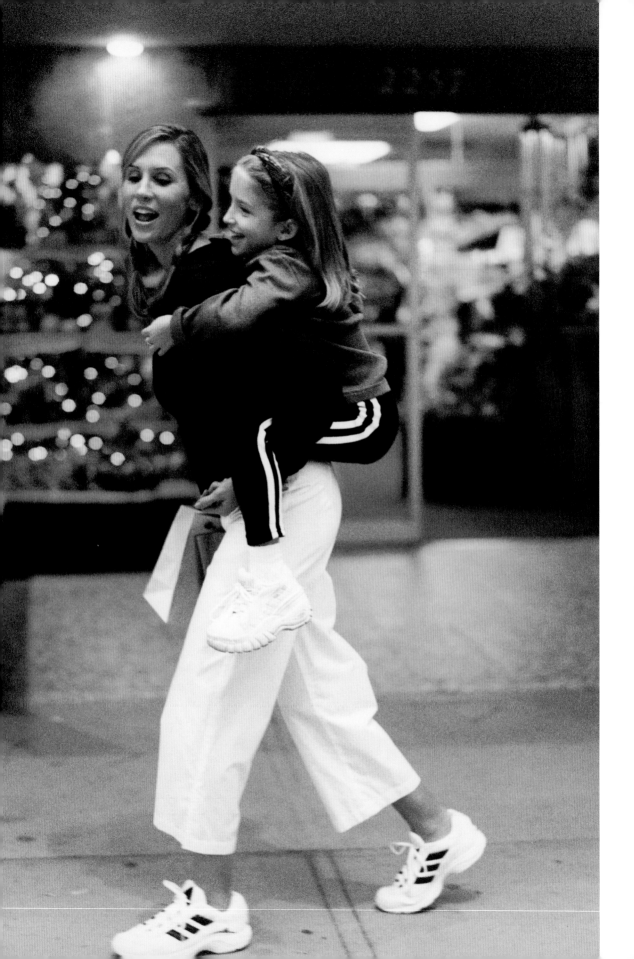

- **Make children rethink the mom-and-pop shuttle service.** The very term *soccer mom* is oxymoronic to me. If you're a mom (or dad) who spends all day driving kids to activities—school, band practice, dance class, and, yes, soccer—you probably spend very little time actually at or involved in soccer, or any other physical activity, for that matter. Yet that's exactly what you need. Take a look at the various places children need to be shuttled day in and day out and try to find ways to spend less time in a car, more on foot or on a bicycle. Could you walk them to a friend's house a few times, teach them a safe route you're comfortable with, and eventually let them go alone? Or could the other parent meet you halfway, so that you both get in a walk? If safety is an issue—say, you can't let them walk to soccer because it finishes after dark—could parents from the neighborhood take turns walking or biking with several kids, helping out at practice, and getting them home safely?

- **Build social activities around being more active.** Backyard barbecue or backyard volleyball? Lying on the beach or walking along the sand? Picnic in the park or playing catch and Frisbee first? The differences are subtle, but they turn sedentary gatherings into opportunities to be active and get others involved.

- **Plan a super-active vacation.** Depending on what you choose, this could be like throwing down the gauntlet: "Who wants to go to the Grand Canyon for vacation?" (Enthusiastic cheers.) "Who wants to actually hike down and see the mighty Colorado River up close?" (Even more cheering.) "And who's ready to get in shape for that hike?" Well, that's the question, and the answer is anybody who wants to have an amazing, life-changing experience. Plan a once-in-a-lifetime vacation and get in shape for it. Then start planning next year's!

Walk Talk: How do I make my neighborhood better for walking? How do I even figure out what's wrong with it?

Lots of people know neighborhoods or streets where they'd never let children walk alone, or where they wouldn't want to walk themselves. But few take the time to ponder, "What makes this place so unwalkable?" It's worth figuring out for two reasons. First, you're never going to be able to fix it until you figure out what's wrong. Second, there actually is money in the federal transportation budget (in fact, one section is called "transportation enhancements") earmarked for improvements to bicycle and pedestrian facilities. So if you know what you're asking for, you might actually get it. And trust me on this—local officials would love to have you help them get some federal dollars into your city or town.

Where do you start? Build public awareness of the need for change or improvements. One way is to talk with friends, neighbors, and other concerned citizens. Another is to distribute and fill out walkability checklists. On page 230 you'll find a very simple one designed to be completed by a parent and child out for a walk together. The best approach is to take a typical walk—to a friend's, a school, the store—and fill out the checklist for your walk. Have others do the same thing, and look for common problems or issues. Then get transportation and elected officials involved and see what you can get fixed. (See the "Walkable Community Information" in the resource list at the end of this book.)

✔ Neighborhood Walkability Checklist*

Take a typical walk in your community—to the store or a friend's house—and answer the five questions below. When answering, check all responses that apply, and be sure to note where you ran into any of the problems that you mention (a street address or cross-street). Then give a general rating from 1 to 6 for each question (1 = awful; 2 = many problems; 3 = some problems; 4 = good; 5 = very good; 6 = excellent).

1. **Did you have room to walk?**
   - ❏ **Yes.**
   - ❏ **No.**

   If no, check all that apply (and note problem locations):
   - ❏ **Sidewalks started and stopped.**
   - ❏ **Sidewalks were broken or cracked.**
   - ❏ **Sidewalks were blocked with poles, signs, Dumpsters, and so on.**
   - ❏ **No sidewalks, paths, or shoulders to walk on.**
   - ❏ **Too much traffic to walk on the side of the road.**

   Anything else? _____

   Rating (1 to 6): _____

2. **Was it easy to cross streets?**
   - ❏ **Yes.**
   - ❏ **No.**

   If no, check all that apply (and note problem locations):
   - ❏ **Road was too wide to get across.**
   - ❏ **Traffic signals made us wait too long, or didn't give enough time to cross.**
   - ❏ **Needed striped crosswalks or traffic signals.**
   - ❏ **Parked cars blocked our view of traffic.**
   - ❏ **Trees or plants blocked our view of traffic.**
   - ❏ **Needed curb ramps, or ramps needed repair.**

   Anything else? _____

   Rating (1 to 6): _____

3. **Did drivers behave well?**
   - ❏ **Yes.**
   - ❏ **No.**

   If no, check all that apply (and note problem locations):

   Drivers . . .
   - ❏ **Backed out of driveways without looking.**
   - ❏ **Did not yield to people crossing.**
   - ❏ **Turned into people crossing streets.**
   - ❏ **Drove too fast.**
   - ❏ **Sped up to make it through traffic lights or drove through red lights.**
   - ❏ **Stopped in or blocked crosswalks.**

   Anything else? _____

   Rating (1 to 6): _____

4. **Did you feel safe?**
   - ❏ **Yes.**
   - ❏ **No.**

   If no, check all that apply (and note problem locations):
   - ❏ **Saw suspicious activity or people.**
   - ❏ **No apparent houses, stores, or other places to go in case of trouble.**
   - ❏ **No public telephones.**

❑ Too dark—lights broken or not present.

❑ Too few other pedestrians—too little activity on the street.

Anything else? _____

Rating (1 to 6): _____

5. **Was it a pleasant place to walk?**

❑ Yes.

❑ No.

If no, check all that apply (and note problem locations):

❑ Needs more grass, flowers, or trees.

❑ Needs water fountains.

❑ Not enough shade.

❑ No benches or places to sit.

❑ Not well lit.

❑ Dirty, lots of litter, trash, graffiti.

❑ No public art or other appealing features.

Anything else? _____

Rating (1 to 6): _____

Add up your score and see how your community did. If you scored:

- **26 to 30.** Celebrate! You have a great neighborhood for walking.

- **21 to 25.** Celebrate a little; your neighborhood is pretty good.

- **16 to 20.** Okay, but it needs work.

- **11 to 15.** It needs a lot of work. Walkers deserve better than this.

- **10 or less.** Call out the National Guard before walking, and start working for change.

If your community scored poorly, you have to take action. First, share your findings with elected officials (for example, the mayor's office or city council) and public services like the departments of public works, transportation, and police. Let the media know about trouble spots. Most important, get out and fix what you can. Here are some simple things you can do (also see "Ten Ways to Spend Your Day Off" at the end of this chapter).

- Organize a neighborhood cleanup day or simply take a bag and pick up trash along your normal walking routes.

- Trim your hedges or trees that might block sidewalks or obscure a pedestrian's view at a crosswalk; ask your neighbors to do the same (or offer to do it for them).

- Be a considerate driver—set an example by driving at safe speeds in neighborhoods, letting pedestrians cross at intersections, and not stopping in crosswalks. Urge family and friends to do the same.

- Notify the animal control officer of scary dogs, and the police of suspicious activity.

- Plant trees and flowers if you have property abutting sidewalks or trails. Or adopt and care for a public space or garden (many towns encourage this) along walking routes.

- Report streetlights or signal lights that are out to the department of public works.

- If you have sidewalk on your property, set an example by quickly clearing it of snow or other debris.

Adapted from the checklist of the Partnership for a Walkable America; see "Walkable Community Information" in the resource list at the end of this book.

Get them walking at work

There are reams of research on work-site wellness and fitness programs, and as you might imagine, starting a walking group is one of the most common "interventions." (That's what public health people call it when they try to improve a community's health; free flu shots are an intervention, for example, as are antismoking campaigns.) Here's what happens: A club is launched, posters are put up, teams are formed, and everyone records their miles. Maybe lunchtime meetings are held with tips on selecting shoes or stretching, and eventually people get T-shirts and coffee mugs for reaching their goals or walking so many days or whatever's required. Then you know what happens? The 10- or 12- or 16-week program ends and most people go back to their old habits. A small fraction may continue walking at lunch or after work, but most slowly drift back to whatever they were or weren't doing before the intervention started. Not a very encouraging picture, eh?

I believe the core problem is that it's just another type of formal exercise. It's a great exercise—my favorite—but if it wasn't part of daily life before the intervention, why would it be afterward? Instead, try an approach that either makes the incentive to walk more permanent than a T-shirt, or makes walking a part of a routine task (like getting to work). Ideally, do both.

Here are a few ideas. Keep in mind that you don't have to make these changes singlehandedly where you work. You may have a benefits manager and wellness coordinator who already know that a more physically active workforce is also healthier and more productive, has lower absenteeism, and requires less health care spending. They simply need help getting people moving. Help them get started by being an example and by helping them with these more creative approaches. (If your company is smaller than this, go straight to management with these ideas.)

- **Encourage walking, transit, and carpools.** Work with management to create incentives to reduce the number of cars in the parking lot. Give employees who actually walk to work, to mass transit, or to a carpool partner's house a break on their health care premium—real money in their pocket, for real money saved by the company. How about an active system of helping employees find coworkers in their community with whom they could carpool? Then encourage them to alternate days walking to one another's house for the ride, rather than getting picked up.

- **Offer parking cash-outs.** A very concrete incentive to getting people out of their cars is to actually give them the cash equivalent of the cost of their parking if they don't drive to work. In some major cities a parking space can cost up to hundreds of dollars a month; sometimes it's provided to employees for free. When it is, those employees who don't use it should get the equivalent in cash—a great incentive. The negative version is to charge an arm and a leg for parking. Dogmatic, perhaps, but it's one reason that 70 percent of Manhattanites don't own cars.

- **Build it into the workday.** In settings where a rigid schedule is required—working on an assembly line, or answering telephone calls—walking breaks can be scheduled into the day. Bonus breaks specifically for walking can even be offered. The schedule may require so many minutes for lunch and morning and afternoon breaks, but you can also allow an additional 10 or 15 minutes for people who will specifically walk during that time. The lost minutes are far outweighed by the increased satisfaction, effectiveness, and health of the employees who choose to walk.

- **Give away some vacation.** How'd you like to earn a day of paid vacation for every 100 miles or 30 hours of walking you log? At some enlightened workplaces you already can. They've realized that active employees are so much healthier and happier that they get lots more done even with some extra days off. Some worksites will let you earn up to an extra week of vacation with your walking.

- **Provide places to walk.** You can't encourage people to walk if there's no place to do it. But the solution can be as mundane as marking the mileage around the perimeter of the parking areas or on nearby sidewalks. Forward-thinking employers are more proactive—building sidewalks, creating trails and nature preserves on their property, and supporting nearby rail-trails (see the Rails-to-Trails Conservancy under "Walkable Community Information" in the resource list).

- **Create friendly competition.** There's no doubt that creating departmental teams and recording mileage can really get people involved. But if you do this, be sure it's encouraging to everyone. Base team-total competitions on time spent walking (this gives fast and slow walkers an equal chance). Hold relay races where ages and abilities are balanced across teams, and everyone's time is added together for the team total. Or hold predicted-time races, where the goal isn't to finish fastest, but to correctly predict how long it will take you to finish a fixed distance. Closest finisher to his prediction wins (no watches allowed, of course). If you insist on the classic walking club approach, at least be clever about it. And make it year-round, not just 10 or 12 weeks.

Ten ways to spend your day off

You've got a weekly plan for walking, and whether you're just shooting for the surgeon general's 30 minutes a day or you're embarking on the training for a sub-six-hour marathon, you'll probably be taking one day a week off from walking. So what are you going to do with all that free time? Before you answer, I have a suggestion: Make the world a friendlier place for walkers. Try any of the following—or, even better, try them all.

1. **Walk with seniors.** Contact a local senior center or elder care facility and volunteer to walk with visitors or residents. Many facilities encourage people to volunteer, and it's possible to offer to help seniors do errands on foot. Most important, of course, can be an opportunity to simply visit while encouraging people to enjoy important physical activity.

2. **Put on a walking event.** Walking events are blossoming in popularity—even running race directors admit that walkers are making up an ever-growing portion of their participants. So if you or your organization would like to put on a walking event in your community, check out the resource list under "Events." Consider the following (contacts are listed under "Clubs and Walking Organizations" and "Events"):

   - Partner with an existing group interested in walking events. If you're thinking of a non-competitive event, contact the American Volkssport Association for your local chapter.

   - If it will be a competitive event, contact your region's racewalking chairperson through USA Track and Field's national office.

   - If your event intends to go big-time, check out the Road Race Management Web site and newsletter.

3. **Build a trail.** The good news is you don't have to do it with your bare hands—although that can actually be the most fun. But this could range from helping to build or maintain a section of rugged, backcountry hiking trail to helping to get a section of old railroad right-of-way turned into a multiuse trail through a city or town. For the former, see the American Hiking Society and other trail organizations under "Hiking" in the resource list. For the latter, contact the Rails-to-Trails Conservancy and regional trail and greenway groups under "Walkable Community Information" in the list. Also, think about organizing locally—

getting neighbors and friends interested in trails in and around your community. This can make you more effective when you approach elected officials for support, property easements, funding, and other necessary steps in creating a trail.

4. **Measure your neighborhood's walkability.** Make copies of the "Neighborhood Walkability Checklist" in this book (see page 230) and hand them out to neighbors, friends, and family. Have people fill them out on typical walks, then collect them and look for common problem areas. Share your findings with city hall and the department of public works, then start to advocate for improvements. Many times facilities are allowed to languish simply because no one has asked for help.

   Also consider handing out the checklist at walking events or to parents and children who routinely walk to school. It can be a useful tool in helping people realize where they're dissatisfied with the walking environment, and start to make changes.

5. **Organize a Walk a Child to School Day.** One of the most exciting walking events happening in the United States and around the world (especially in England and Canada) is International Walk a Child to School Day. The idea is simple—parents, caregivers, and children are encouraged to walk to school on this one day (usually during the first week in October) to recognize the need for safe, accessible walking routes and the importance of daily activity for kids. (Children are at the same risks for inactivity as adults in America; childhood obesity rates have skyrocketed in the past 30 years!) But this is more than a one-day event.

   The fundamental idea is to encourage children to walk every day, not just on Walk to School Day. Communities have improved crosswalks, hired crossing guards, launched safety education programs, and repaired sidewalks and pathways as a result of feedback from adults and kids during Walk to School events. Many schools distribute walkability checklists so that walkers can catalog opportunities for improvement during their walks.

6. **Start a walking school bus.** You've had a Walk to School Day, but how do you keep the kids (and adults) walking? By launching a walking school bus, of course. Conceived in the United Kingdom and Canada, this idea is rapidly spreading around cities in the United States. The notion is to create standard routes that children will walk to school with adult supervision. As the "bus" walks along the route (sometimes the adults wear colored hats or scarves), children are picked up along the way. Often parents set up a schedule to share the driver duty—I'll take Monday, you on Tuesday, and so on. It's even common for the adults to pull a wagon for the children's book bags, to make the walking easier for the kids (and a better workout for Mom or Dad!).

   This has the immense advantage of keeping kids walking year-round—the "walking buses" are even successful in cold-weather cities such as Chicago and Toronto—while allaying parents' safety concerns. Children are taught safe pedestrian behaviors, and the environment becomes safer simply because there are more people out on the street.

7. **Show up at planning board meetings.** Many of the most important decisions regarding the walkability of your community are made at the local level. How your local planning and zoning board allocates open space, whether it requires sidewalks in new neighborhoods, where schools are built, and the location of commercial centers all have a vast impact on whether you can walk as a part of your daily life. You won't often walk to a corner store to buy milk if the "corner store" is 5 miles away, and that's just what happens if many modern zoning codes are strictly adhered to.

Most zoning codes assume that a separation of uses is good, dating from a time when our industries were filthy and we didn't want their pollution where we lived. But now having the places where we work, live, shop, and play distant from one another requires that we do everything by car. In fact, the U.S. Department of Transportation says that on average, 90 percent or more of all trips from home are by car!

You have to speak up if you want this to change. Show up at planning meetings and demand that new developments have sidewalks and be zoned to include corner stores and services within walking distance of homes. Insist that schools be built within walking distance of as many of the children they will serve as possible. Advocate for the preservation of open space and linear parks with pathways and trails to connect neighborhoods, schools, and commercial areas. Rest assured that your voice will be heard. I've gotten involved in my town and been surprised to see how few people actually show up and speak up at such public meetings—yet those who do have a substantial influence on the process.

8. **Talk to candidates, write to Congress, vote.** Federal legislation and state budgets can have a huge impact on you as a walker. Recent federal transportation budgets (the most recent is TEA-21, the Transportation Equity Act for the 21st Century) earmarked a small fraction of their funds specifically for bicycle, pedestrian, and transit programs and facilities. Since the total budgets are hundreds of *billions* of dollars over several years, this still leaves hundreds of millions for use by each state to fund bicycle and pedestrian trails, safety improvements, transit systems, and more.

We must all vocally advocate both putting these dollars to work benefiting pedestrians and bicyclists within our states and increasing this use of our tax dollars. It's clear that simply building more roads isn't going to solve our congestion, pollution, or energy consumption problems, and it doesn't help our public health at all. Eventually, however, having a lot more Americans walk and bike to the store or work could make a difference on these pressing issues. Let your national and state legislators know that you don't want pedestrians to be forgotten!

9. **Look for a new house—live where you can walk!** What I mean is that you should look for a community where you can walk more and drive less. Consider living in a place where 9 out of 10 times you step out the front door to go somewhere you don't have to start the car—you can simply walk or bicycle where you want to go. This means choosing a community where school, work, shopping, and play are all within walking distance.

Does this sound crazy? Well, think for a moment about some of the most desirable cities and towns in America—places that regularly rank high on published lists of America's most livable communities. One of the universal elements in these places—from Portland, Maine, to Portland, Oregon, and from Madison, Wisconsin, to Austin, Texas—is that they are built on a human scale, and they invite you to be out and about on foot. Even great cities like Chicago, Boston, and Washington, D.C., have the statuary and landmarks and parks and pathways that encourage rather than discourage walking. The same holds true for the places we choose to go on vacation, from Nantucket to England—one reason we go is because we can walk there and enjoy it!

The more you preserve places like these and move to places like them, the more you convince developers, chambers of commerce, and elected officials that maybe this is what all cities and towns should be like. So you not only make your own life more walkable, you make a strong statement by your choice.

Large cities.

Boston, MA.	Lots of pre-automobile history—nearly 400 years' worth—and growth constrained by water on three sides assured Boston took on a compact, magnificently walkable form.
Chicago, IL.	A little wind doesn't keep Chicagoans in droves away from the Lakeshore path; it's ideal for walking, cycling, in-line skating, and especially people-watching. A traditional grid and fine transit make Chicago inviting.
Minneapolis, MN.	A city laced with trails and bike lanes, many connecting the green space surrounding the city's innumerable lakes. Car-free Nicolette Boulevard and downtown residential redevelopment further boost the appeal for the actively inclined.
New York, NY.	The city may never sleep, but it sure does walk a lot. Every block is a walker's delight to explore—you never know what type of restaurant, shop, or street vendor you'll stumble on next—and New York is building a world-class greenway system.
Portland, OR.	A pedestrianized downtown, a growing network of bike lanes and pathways, and mixed-use development that encourages neighborhoods where life, work, and play are all within walking distance are the results of decades' worth of policy effort.
San Francisco, CA.	The hills only enhance the appeal of strolling the City by the Bay. Myriad colorful neighborhoods and a walkable waterfront all the way to the Presidio—a former military base turned beautiful urban park—beg exploration on foot.
Seattle, WA.	You feel the outdoor ethic of the region as you circle Green Lake or wander the pedestrian-friendly neighborhoods throughout the city; the Burke-Gilman trail is a nonmotorized spine that sets the standard for urban trails nationwide.
Washington, DC.	Laid out as an easily navigated grid with angled boulevards connecting grand civic buildings and creating scores of inviting public circles and pocket parks, plus a great subway system, still-growing trail network, and more national monuments than you can shake a stick at.

Medium-size cities.

Arlington, VA.	Transit-oriented development makes it easy to live without a car in this Washington, D.C., suburb.
Boulder, CO.	One of America's first car-free zones, Pearl Street mall, is still one of the best, along with great trails, transit, and pedestrian boulevards.
Burlington, VT.	Walk the waterfront trail along Lake Champlain, and explore the downtown pedestrian zone.

Cambridge, MA.	A network of bike lanes, the Charles River waterfront trail, and great walkable neighborhoods.	
Chattanooga, TN.	Saving the bridge at Walnut Street for bicyclists and pedestrians stimulated a riverfront trail system and downtown revival.	
Davis, CA.	A conscious effort to keep the city from being overrun by cars begun 30 years ago has made this America's bicycling capital!	
Lincoln, NE.	A growing trail system and traditional downtown grid boost walking in this university town.	
Madison,WI.	State Street is always full of bikes and pedestrians, as are the trails around the city's lakes.	
Mt. Lebanon, PA.	So committed to walkable, neighborhood schools that no child is bused to school.	
Portland, ME.	Great waterfront walking defines this inviting New England port city, including the inner harbor area.	
Santa Barbara, CA.	Walk the oceanfront trail to the college or to kayak, surf, fine outdoor dining, or just to walk; then bike up to the historic Mission.	
West Palm Beach, FL.	A model of urban redevelopment that used walkability as a central tenet of the economic rebirth.	

Smaller cities and towns. (Just a sampling of the hundreds across the US!)

Alexandria, VA	Crested Butte, CO	Livingston, MO
Annapolis, MD	Dunedin, FL	Portsmouth, NH
Arcata, CA	Exeter, NH	Saratoga Springs, NY
Brockport, NY	Fort Collins, CO	Savannah, GA
Charleston, SC	Glenwood Springs, CO	Traverse City, MI
Chautauqua, NY	Jackson, WY	Xenia, OH

10. **Be a role model—go for a walk.** And so I end where I began—urging you to simply head out the door and go for a walk. Because this is truly what it's all about. When you walk, you improve yourself—but you also improve your community. By your mere presence outside, enjoying one of life's simplest and healthiest activities, you invite others to join you. You change the landscape simply by being there, suggesting to others that maybe it's worth heading out and taking a walk. Which, of course, is something you already know.

Resources

APPAREL

These Web sites and catalogs are good one-stop resources for athletic clothing from a variety of companies.

www.lucy.com: Women's exercise apparel, shoes, equipment, and accessories; call 877-WWW-LUCY (877-999-5829) for a mail-order catalog.

www.fogdog.com: Men's and women's apparel, shoes, equipment, and accessories; no mail-order catalogs are available, but you can call 800-624-2017 for customer service or to place an order.

www.walkingshop.com; www.roadrunnersports.com: Tons of shoes, plus apparel and gear, reviews, and discounts; call 800-636-3560 for a mail-order catalog or to place an order.

BABY BACKPACKS

See "Child Carriers"

BACKPACKING and CAMPING

See "Hiking"

BICYCLING (MOUNTAIN BIKING)

Bicycle manufacturers and especially bike shops are great sources of information about where and how to get started biking.

International Mountain Bicycling Association: Environmentally and socially responsible mountain biking. Call 888-442-IMBA (888-442-4622) or check out www.imba.com to find leaders near you and membership information.

CHILD CARRIERS

Prices may vary according to location.

Baby Bjorn: 866-424-0200; www.babybjorn.com. Offers eight fabric choices for its soft front carriers ($88).

Kelty: 800-423-2320 (Canada 800-361-0377); www.kelty.com. Soft and frame carriers available from retailers nationwide ($50 to $260).

Tough Traveler: 800-GO-TOUGH (800-468-6844); www.toughtraveler.com. Soft and frame carriers available; can order by phone or online ($90 to $170).

Evenflo: 800-233-5921 (Canada 800-265-0749); www.evenflo.com. Snugli soft and frame carriers available through retailers nationwide ($20 to $100).

Some Helpful Web Sites

www.babygear.com: Find discounts on several brands, plus product reviews.

www.barronmall.com: Offers discounted Kelty baby carriers and other products that allow you to hike more comfortably with your child.

CLUBS and WALKING ORGANIZATIONS

American Volkssport Association
1001 Pat Booker Road
Suite 101, Phoenix Square
Universal City, TX 78148-4147
Phone: 800-830-WALK (800-830-9255)
Web site: www.ava.org

AVA's 500 clubs organize more than 3,000 noncompetitive events per year nationwide. Call or visit the Web site to find a club or event near you.

American Walking Association
P.O. Box 20491
Boulder, CO 80308-3491
Web site: www.walking.about.com

Call to find coaches, camps, and clinics across the country. For a free informational kit, including facts about the organization, safety tips, and a shoe-buying guide, send a business-size self-addressed stamped envelope to the above address.

YMCA
888-333-YMCA (888-333-9622); www.ymca.com
The nation's largest not-for-profit community service organization. Many communities offer walking programs; for information about specific programs, call your local YMCA.

www.walking.about.com/sports/walking/msubrwcl.htm: Links to Web sites of national and regional walking and racewalking clubs.

www.surf.to/worldclass: Coach Dave McGovern's Web page with links to walking, racewalking, and walker-friendly running clubs.

Also see the North American Racewalking Foundation under "Racewalking."

EVENTS (Walking Events, Organizers, and Information)

American Diabetes Association's Step Out to Fight Diabetes Walks (formerly called Team Diabetes Walks: 1-800-DIABETES. Walk or run a marathon (26.2 miles). *Minimum donation is $3,000 to $4,000, depending on your choice of location: Chicago, Disney World, Dublin, Las Vegas, Kona, Maui, San Francisco, Rome, Quebec, Ottawa, or Vancouver.*

American Heart Association (AHA): 800-AHA-USA1 (800-242-8721);
go to www.americanheart.org and search for "American Heart Walk"
American Heart Walk is the AHA's premier walking and fund-raising event that takes place in over 1,000 cities every year. This noncompetitive event typically occurs on the last weekend of September or first weekend of October.

Arthritis Foundation's Joints in Motion Event: 1-877-9JOINTS; www.arthritis.org
Walk or run a marathon (26.2 miles). Airfare, hotels, and entry fees are covered if you meet your fund-raising goal. Minimum pledges range from $2,500 to $5,000, depending on your choice of location: New Orleans, Vancouver, Dublin, or Honolulu.

Avon 3-Day Breast Cancer Walks: 1-800-510-WALK; www.avoncrusade.com
Sixty-mile group walks including food, tent accommodations, and entertainment. Minimum pledge $1,800. Event locations: Atlanta, Boston, Chicago, Los Angeles, New York, San Francisco, and Washington, D.C.

International Marching League (IML) Walking Association: (+31) 24 365-5500; www.imwalking.org/
Oversees 20- to 50-kilometer multiday walks in great locations around the world.

Leukemia Society of America Marathons: 800-482-TEAM (800-482-8326); www.teamintraining.org
Walk or run a marathon (26.2 miles). Airfare, hotels, and entry fees are covered if you meet your fund-raising goal. Minimum pledge varies with event; there are more than 30 events in this series.

March of Dimes WalkAmerica: 800-525-WALK (800-525-9255) January through April; 914-428-7100 year-round; www.walkamerica.org
The March of Dimes' biggest fund raiser, WalkAmerica supports lifesaving research and community programs that save babies from birth defects, low birthweight, and infant death. WalkAmerica will take place in 1,400 communities in all 50 states, the District of Columbia, and Puerto Rico. In most communities WalkAmerica is held at the end of April. Routes vary in length, but most are about 20 kilometers (approximately 12 miles).

MS Walk: 800-FIGHT-MS (800-344-4867); www.nmss.org
The MS Walk will be offered in 700 cities across the nation, with distances from 3 to 12 miles; accessible routes are always available. Complimentary food, beverages, first aid, and special transportation provided.

Road Race Management: 301-320-6865; www.rrm.com
A Web site and newsletter dedicated to the work of directing successful road races.

Race for the Cure: 972-855-1600 or 888-603-RACE (888-603-7223)
Fax: 972-855-1605
Web site: www.raceforthecure.com

The Komen Race for the Cure series has become the largest series of 5K and 1-mile run/fitness walks in the nation, held in 108 cities across the country in 2000 with over a million participants expected. Proceeds fund both national research efforts and local breast cancer initiatives.

USA Track and Field: 317-261-0500; www.racewalk.com
The national governing body for track and field (including racewalking) in the United States. The national office can connect you with your local chapter and local racewalking chair, and provide a calendar of events.

Walk a Child to School Day: The goal is for children, parents and community leaders to walk to school together with a purpose—to promote safety, health, physical activity and concern for the environment. See contact information under "International Walk a Child to School Day."

Athletic Footwear

Most of the companies below have online catalogs and store-finder features on their Web sites.

www.roadrunnersports.com: A one-stop Web site for many different brands, plus reviews and discounts; call 800-636-3560 for a mail-order catalog.

Adidas: 800-448-1796; www.adidas.com. Create your own training schedule; read about star athletes; download screen savers, wallpapers, and games online.

Asics: 800-678-9435; www.asicsamerica.com. Web site lists upcoming events and promotions, answers some technical questions.

Avia: 888-855-AVIA (888-855-2842); www.aviashoes.com. Web site features a short article and workout program by a fitness expert.

Easy Spirit: 888-EASY-772 (888-327-9772); www.easyspirit.com. Call to find retailers, ask questions.

New Balance: 800-253-SHOE (800-253-7463); www.newbalance.com. Online calendar of running and walking events nationwide.

Nike: 800-344-6453; www.nike.com. Online Nike iD feature allows you to build your own shoes.

Puma: 800-662-PUMA (800-662-7862); www.puma.com. Check out newsworthy athletes and download games or a soundtrack from the Web site.

Reebok: 800-843-4444; www.reebok.com. Access information on Reebok's several brands, recommended workouts, and an exercise log for recording progress.

Ryka: 888-834-RYKA (888-834-7952); www.ryka.com. Web site offers workout tips for women.

Saucony: 800-365-7282; www.saucony.com. Web site offers workout tips.

Teva: 800-FOR-TEVA (800-367-8382); www.teva.com. Men's and women's sport-specific performance sandals, including a new running sandal.

Rugged Footwear

These shoes and boots are more suited to the trail; also see hiking outfitters.

Hi-Tec: 800-521-1698; www.hi-tec.com

L.L. Bean: 800-221-4221; www.llbean.com

Merrell: 800-789-8586; www.merrellboot.com

Montrail: 800-249-1642; www.montrail.com

North Face: 866-715-3223; www.thenorthface.com

Rockport: 888-ROCKPORT (888-762-5767); www.rockport.com

Tecnica: 800-258-3897; www.tecnicausa.com

Timberland: 800-445-5545; www.timberland.com

Vasque: 800-224-HIKE (800-224-4453); www.vasque.com

HEART-RATE MONITORS

Creative Health Products: 800-742-4478; www.chponline.com. Discounted health products—free information, catalog, and pricing when you call.

CardioSport: 888-760-3059; www.cardiosport.com. All monitors are water-resistant to 20 meters and have handlebar adapters for use on indoor fitness equipment.

Polar: 800-227-1314; www.polarusa.com. Waterproof, long battery life. Personal trainer, coaching tips, and special events sections on Web page.

Acumen: 800-852-7823; www.acumeninc.com. Acumen Basix Plus model monitors heart rate and even calculates your target range.

HIKING: Contacts, Information, and Outdoor Outfitters

Hiking Organizations

American Hiking Society: 301-565-6704; www.americanhiking.org. A national hiking and trail advocacy organization, which can help you get in touch with a club in your area.

Appalachian Mountain Club: 617-523-0636; www.outdoors.org. America's oldest conservation and recreation organization, based in the northeastern United States. The AMC teaches skills, operates lodges, fixes trails, publishes guides, and works on conservation issues.

Sierra Club: 415-977-5500; www.sierraclub.org. This well-known environmental organization provides information on current environmental issues, teaches conservation skills, and sponsors hundreds of national and international outings per year.

Books

50 Hikes series, by Backcountry Publications/Countryman Press
P.O. Box 748
Woodstock, VT 05091
Phone: 800-245-4151
Web site: www.countrymanpress.com/series/50-hikes.html
More than 20 books in the series cover the northeastern United States, as well as Ohio, Michigan, North Carolina, Tennessee, and Virginia.

Ultimate Guide to Backcountry Travel, by Michael Lanza (Appalachian Mountain Club Books, 1999): Loads of information on everything from packing to using a compass to coping with wild animals, presented in an enjoyable and readable package. Visit www.outdoors.org, or call 800-262-4455.

The Essential Guide to Hiking in the United States, by Charles Cook (Michael Kesend Publishing, 1991): Provides a state-by-state listing of hiking areas, the governing bodies (and their addresses), the best hiking areas and trails, and a description of the areas and the wildlife and flora to be found. Visit amazon.com or Barns&Noble.com

FalconGuides® series, including state-specific guides and the *Best Easy Day Hikes* series (www.globepequot.com)

Maps

National Geographic: 800-NGS-LINE (800-647-5463); www.ngstore.com

A wide selection of hiking and recreation maps is also available, including *Complete Trail Smart: National Parks of the USA*, a five-CD set ($99).

Rand McNally: 847-329-8100; www.randmcnally.com

Download and print maps for all 50 states, as well as more than 30 thematic maps.

U.S. Geological Survey: 888-ASK-USGS (888-275-8747); mapping.usgs.gov/

View maps online before ordering.

Trail Organizations

Appalachian Trail Conference (East Coast): 304-535-6331; www.appalachiantrail.org

Continental Divide Trail Alliance (Rocky Mountain States): 888-909-CDTA (888-909-2382); www.cdtrail.org

East Coast Greenway Alliance: Overseeing completion of a nonmotorized trail from Maine to Florida through all of the major cities of the eastern seaboard; www.greenway.org

North Country Trail Association (Great Lakes and Upper Midwest): 1-866-HIKENCT (866-445-3628; www.northcountrytrail.org/

American Discovery Trail Society (Delaware to California): 800-663-2387; www.discoverytrail.org

Lewis and Clark Trail: The National Park Service publishes and distributes a general information brochure and map of the trail, free of charge, to help with trip planning. For a copy of the general brochure, contact the NPS at 402-661-1804 or visit www.nps.gov/lecl for information on how to contact visitor centers along the trail.

Pacific Crest Trail Association: 888-PCTRAIL (888-728-7245); www.pcta.org

Outdoor Outfitters and Other Great Resources

Mail-Order Catalogs

L.L. Bean: Call 800-441-5713 to request a catalog or visit www.llbean.com for clothing and gear, plus an international park search feature.

Recreational Equipment, Inc. (REI): Call 800-426-4840 to request a catalog, or visit www.rei.com for the gear shop, a learn and share feature, classes and events, plus a link to the REI outlet store.

Web Sites

camping.about.com: A wealth of information on outdoor gear, services, clubs, and organizations, plus links to related sites.

www.altrec.com: Plenty of gear offerings, plus a how-to-buy feature. Links to other sports, such as cycling, climbing, paddling, and snow sports. Live online service, or call 800-369-3949.

www.kidssource.com: This Web site caters to active outdoor families, providing information and gear for parents and children, and helpful links to related sites.

www.greatoutdoors.com: Gear, weather, recipes, and tips for a variety of outdoor sports.

www.gorp.com: Plan a trip, buy gear and maps, read tips and articles about outdoor activities, find or rate a trail, or post a message on the discussion boards.

www.4hiking.com: Gear, tips, trails and tours, and links to related sites, such as hiking and trail organizations.

www.planetoutdoors.com: Wide selection of gear, plus tips and articles.

www.backroads.com: To plan an outdoor vacation, visit the Web site or call 800-GO-ACTIVE (800-462-2848).

ICE

These products may aid with icing after an injury. Most are available through your local pharmacy.

Aircast Cryo/Cuff: 800-336-6569; go to www.aircast.com/help/sitemap.htm. Click on Product Information for Cryo/Cuff

BD Ace Cold Therapy Products: www.bd.com/elastics/index1.asp

Contour Pak: 800-926-2228; www.contourpak.com

Thera-Med Cold Pack: 800-327-7845; www.thera-med.com

INSTRUCTORS and INSTRUCTOR CERTIFICATION

Instructor and personal trainer certification groups.

Aerobics and Fitness Association of America (AFAA)
15250 Ventura Boulevard
Suite 200
Sherman Oaks, CA 91403
1-877-YOUR-BODY (1-877-968-7263)
Fax: 818-788-6301
Web site: www.afaa.com

American College of Sports Medicine (ACSM)
P.O. Box 1440
Indianapolis, IN 46206-1440
Phone: 317-637-9200
Fax: 317-634-7817
Web site: www.acsm.org

American Council on Exercise (ACE)
4851 Paramount Drive
San Diego, CA 92123
Phone: 858-279-8227 or 888-825-3636
Fax: 858-279-8064
Web site: www.acefitness.org

IDEA (the international association of fitness professionals)
Phone: 800-999-4332, ext. 7
Fax: 858-535-8234
Web site: www.ideafit.com

Racewalking Instructors

Dave McGovern; members.aol.com/rayzwocker/worldclass/clinics.htm

A former member of the U.S. National Racewalking Team, Dave now coaches walkers of all levels and hosts Dave's World Class Racewalking Clinics around the country. Look for his books, The Complete Guide to Racewalking *and* The Complete Guide to Walking a Marathon, *or contact him about clinics in your area.*

Bonnie Stein: www.acewalker.com

Bonnie runs her Ace Walker programs of instruction, coaching, and personal training with an infectious style and deep passion for walking. She teaches everyone how to racewalk—some choose to compete, others walk for health and fitness, and many walk with weight loss as a goal.

INTERNATIONAL WALK A CHILD TO SCHOOL DAY

This national observance encourages children, parents, and community leaders to walk to school together with a purpose—to promote safety, health, physical activity, and concern for the environment. The ultimate goal is to create a more walkable world community by community. Normally scheduled around the first Wednesday in October.

www.walktoschool-usa.org (U.S. information)

www.iwalktoschool.org (international information)

www.saferoutesinfo.org (now to launch a comprehensive Safe Routes to School program)

KAYAKS

There are many manufacturers of kayaks, but here are some that offer nice lines of introductory and recreational craft. It's best to find a dealer in your area who has demonstrations on local waters. Your best bet is to try renting a few times before you buy.

Old Town: 207-827-5514; www.otccanoe.com

Wilderness Systems: 800-59KAYAK (800-595-2925); www.wildernesssystems.org

Seaward Kayaks: 800-595-9755; www.seawardkayaks.com

Necky Kayaks: 800-8-KAYAKS; www.necky.com

Kokatat: 800-225-9749; www.kokatat.com. For all manner of paddling information, apparel, and PFDs (personal flotation devices), including jackets, pants, wet and dry suits, plus supplemental safety gear.

MALL WALKING

WalkSport America: 800-757-WALK (800-757-9255); www.walksport.com. This organization sponsors a national mall-walking program called WalkSport, which has swipe cards for use in member malls around the country. To locate member malls, call or visit the Web site.

ORIENTEERING

U.S. Orienteering Federation: 404-363-2110; www.us.orienteering.org. They can help you learn about local events and clubs in your area.

PEDOMETERS

For greatest accuracy, I recommend pedometers manufactured by Yamax, in Japan. In a comparative research study, they were shown to be highly accurate and consistent from one workout to the next. Here are three manufacturers; the first two distributors use the manufacturer's name for the pedometers, Digi-walkers.

NEW Lifestyles: 888-SIT-LESS (888-748-5377) or 816-353-1852; www.digiwalker.com.

Optimal Health Products: 888-339-2067.

Accusplit: 800-935-1996; www.accusplit.com. They call the same products the Accusplit Eagle series.

POLES, Walking

Exel: 802-846-5565; www.nordicwalker.com. Includes contact information for instructors nationwide.

Exerstrider: 888-285-7392; www.exerstrider.com. Poles, an instructional video, and a manual are available.

Leki: 800-255-9982, www.leki.com. Range of models and prices for different needs. Web site offers a dealer locator feature.

RACEWALKING

USA Track and Field
One RCA Dome, Suite 140
Indianapolis, IN 46225
Phone: 317-261-0500
Fax: 317-261-0481
Web site: www.racewalk.com

The national governing body for track and field and racewalking in the United States. To find your regional track and field office, which can connect you with your local racewalking chairperson and contacts for local walking clubs, contact the national office.

See also "Instructors, Racewalking."

REFLECTIVE PRODUCTS

A safety must for walking after dark.

The Reflectory
P.O. Box 1031
Newburgh, NY 12551
Phone: 845-565-2037
Web site: www.safetyreflectors.com

Free catalog of reflective products and other safety materials.

3M Scotchlite: 888-3M-HELPS (888-364-3577); www.3m.com

illumiNITE: 508-231-0748; www.illuminite.com

PolyBrite: 800-320-3801; www.goeken.com/ipt/index.htm

Stridelite: 425-398-4199; www.stridelite.com

ROCK CLIMBING

Both of the following organizations offer instruction and guided outings throughout the United States, not just for rock climbing but also for a wide variety of outdoor activities including hiking, backpacking, bicycling, kayaking and canoeing, and skiing.

National Outdoor Leadership School (NOLS): 307-332-5300 or 800-710-NOLS (800-710-6657; www.nols.edu/NOLSHome.html. Request a course catalog.

Outward Bound: 888-88-BOUND (888-882-6863); www.outwardbound.org. Request a course catalog.

SNOWSHOES, SNOWSHOEING

These manufacturers have good reputations for providing high-quality snowshoes at reasonable prices, and models suited for both beginners and backcountry travelers.

Atlas Snowshoes, San Francisco: 888-48-ATLAS or 866-747-7013 in Canada; www.atlassnowshoe.com

Crescent Moon, Boulder, Colorado: 800-587-7655; www.crescentmoonsnowshoes.com

Redfeather Snowshoes, Denver: 800-525-0081, www.redfeather.com

Tubbs Snowshoes, Stowe, Vermont: 800-882-2748; www.tubbssnowshoes.com

SOCKS

One of the most mundane pieces of gear, yet one of the most important to a walker. You'll never regret making the investment in quality socks. Here are some brands I've found comfortable and durable over the years, but there are many others as well.

Fox River: 800-247-1815; www.foxrivermills.com. Athletic, outdoor, and winter socks and liners.

Smart Wool: 800-550-WOOL (800-550-9665); www.smartwool.com. Made of natural wool fibers. Socks and liners are available in sport-specific, outdoor, and casual styles.

Thor•Lo: 888-THORLOS (888-846-7567); www.thorlo.com. Sport-specific, outdoor, or casual socks.

Bridgedale: www.bridgedale.com. Sport-specific, durable socks for rugged activities.

STRETCHING

Here are three great resources on different types of stretching, from three highly regarded experts. All are available through any major bookseller.

Shelter Publications, Inc.
P.O. Box 279
Bolinas, CA 94924
415-868-0280
Web site: www.shelterpub.com

Stretching, by Bob Anderson (Shelter Publications, 1980): Easy to use, very simple with clear illustrations, it is the definitive handbook on static stretching for just about any activity.

Facilitated Stretching: PNF Stretching Made Easy, second edition, by Robert McAtee (Human Kinetics Publishers, 1999): A very understandable description of Proprioceptive Neuromuscular Facilitation, with stretches for partners or done alone. Visit www.human kinetics.com.

The Whartons' Stretch Book, by Jim and Phil Wharton (Random House, 1996): This is the definitive manual on Active-Isolated Stretching, by its developers. Call 212-782-9000 or visit www.randomhouse.com.

STROLLERS, All-Terrain

Prices may vary according to location.

Baby Jogger: 800-241-1848; www.babyjogger.com. Choose from eight models, including double, triple, and special-needs strollers. Web site has link to factory outlet ($159.95 to $509).

Baby Trend: 800-328-7363; www.babytrend.com. Offers jogging, tandem, and stand-on strollers, as well as more traditional models. Check Web site for retailers ($160 to $220).

BOB: 800-893-2447; www.bobstrollers.com. Three models of sport-utility strollers ($279 to $399).

Instep: 800-242-6110; www.instep.net. Two stroller models fold up into backpacks; frame carriers also available. Check Web site for retailers.

Kool Stop: 800-247-9754; www.koolstop.com. Choose from four regular models and one special-needs model of Kool-Stride jogging strollers ($249 to $395).

TREADMILLS

Prices may vary according to location.

Cybex: 888-GO-CYBEX; www.ecybex.com. Some models have preprogrammed workouts; some have contact heart-rate monitoring features ($2,985 to $7,995).

PaceMaster: 973-276-9700; www.pacemaster.com. Soft Step impact absorption system; built in warm-up and cool-down functions ($1,795 to $1,995).

Precor: 800-4-PRECOR (800-477-3267); www.precor.com. Most have preprogrammed workouts; some with heart-rate speed controls ($900 to $5,000).

Schwinn: 800-SCHWINN; www.schwinn.com. Most models have preset and user-designed program settings. The 5450p model folds up to save space ($899 to $1,799).

True: 800-426-6570; www.truefitness.com. S.O.F.T. Select system offers advanced shock absorption. Target heart-rate controls; most models are programmable ($1,795 to $5,100).

VESTS, Weight

Ironwear Fitness: 800-630-2779 or 412-782-2212. Vests come in various weights and prices ($99.00 to $379.99). The Uni-Vest™ is the only weight vest line to be endorsed and sold by Reebok™.

X2 Vest Weight Vests by Xtreme Worldwide Athletic Equipment: 800-697-5658. Vests come in 12-pound styles. An additional 8 pounds can be added to increase the total weight to 20 pounds. Cost is $129.99 plus shipping for the 12-pound vest; $20.00 for the additional 8-pound weights.

V-Max Weight Vest by Weight Vest: 208-356-7513. Vests come in 15 pounds and up. Weights can be taken out but not added. Cost is $129.95 (price includes shipping).

Walk Vest: 877-WALKVEST. Vest comes with 8 half-pound weights and can be loaded up to 16 pounds. Cost is $79.95 plus $14.95 shipping for the 4-pound vest. Additional weights sold in 4-pound packages are $14.95 plus $6.95 shipping.

Smart Vest, by Training Zone Concepts, Inc.: 888-797-8378. Weight is adjustable from one pound on up; custom-fit men's and women's models available (black). Cost is $149 with 10-pound weight and training program.

WALK A CHILD TO SCHOOL DAY

See listing for "International Walk a Child to School Day."

WALKABLE COMMUNITY INFORMATION

This is a select list of resources for more livable communities.

Active Living by Design program of the Robert Wood Johnson Foundation, Chapel Hill, NC; www.activelivingbydesign.org. Extensive research bibliography online.

AmericaWalks, Boston, MA; www.americawalks.org. A coalition of about 50 local and regional pedestrian advocacy groups nationwide, provides technical assistance.

Association of Pedestrian and Bicycle Professionals (APBP); www.apbp.org.

Bikes Belong Coalition, Ltd., Brookline, MA: 617-734-2800; www.bikesbelong.org.

Coalition of bicycle industry supporters of more livable community efforts.

Centers for Disease Control and Prevention. www.cdc.gov/nccdphp/dnpa. A site with lots of current data on health and physical activity, and promotional resources.

League of American Bicyclists, Washington, DC, 202-822-1333; www.bikeleague.org. National advocacy group advancing the Bike Friendly Communities program.

Local Government Commission, Sacramento, CA: 916-448-1198; www.lgc.org. Huge library of practical planning and transportation guides; for example, "Real Towns."

National Center for Bicycling and Walking, Washington, D.C; www.bikewalk.org. Provides Walkable Community Workshops, technical assistance, Pro Walk/Pro Bike conference.

Pedestrian and Bicycle Information Center, Chapel Hill, NC.: 877-WALKBIKE; 202-463-8405; www.walkinginfo.org; www.bicyclinginfo.org. Technical support for communities, including walkability and bike-ability checklists and bike/ped facility design guides.

Rails-to-Trails Conservancy, Washington, DC.; www.railtrails.org. Great help for trail and greenway advocates, including research supporting trails' benefits.

Rivers and Trails Conservation Assistance, a program of the National Park Service; www.ncrc.nps.gov/rtca. Provides technical support.

Safe Routes to School programs: www.saferoutesinfo.org. Walk to School day is first Wednesday in October; site has event registry, walking school bus information, extensive resources, and links.

Surface Transportation Policy Project, Washington, D.C. 202-466-2636, www.transact.org. Publishes annual reports loaded with pedestrian activity and safety data.

Victoria Transportation Policy Institute, Victoria, British Columbia; www.vtpi.org. White papers, research evidence, and resources to support alternative transportation..

Walkable Communities, Inc., High Springs, FL: www.walkable.org. The consulting firm of Dan Burden, one of the nation's leading experts.

WATER HYDRATION SYSTEMS

Aquifer vest by Ultimate Direction: 800-426-7229; www.ultimatedirection.com

Back- and waist-worn packs by Camelbak: 800-767-8725; www.camelbak.com/

WEIGHTS, Hand

Healthy Lifestyle Corporation: 310-372-7999; www.energyfirst.com. "Heavy Hands" weights available in four-pound ($24.95 for weights only) and nine-pound ($43.75 for weights only). Handles and an instructional video are also available, and the Web site has photographs of proper technique.

Index to Walk Talks

Answers to common questions about walking. (The Walk Talks.)

Index

recommendations for, 131

self-assessments of, 135–37, 160–61

flashlights, 8

flexibility, 16, 170–71

food guide pyramids, 13, 74

food intake, 10, 71, 73–78

football, 174–75

footwear

hiking, 4, 5, 83, 97, 125–26

injury prevention and, 207, 211

running, 123–24, 162

walking, 4–5, 83, 107, 123–27, 162

Four-Week Warm-Up Program, 3, 4

FPGT (fasting plasma glucose tests), 15

friction, 98

fruits, 74, 75, 77, 78

fund-raising walks, 189–90

gardening, 18

garlic, 77

gear. *See* equipment and gear

gloves, 56

glucose levels, 15

goal setting

national requirements for physical activity, 9

rewards and, 80, 181, 220

for walking, 16, 38, 39, 52, 217–19

Gore-Tex, 55, 104

groups, walking, 38

hamstrings, 43, 208, 210, 211

handball, 174

hand weights, 119

hats, 55–56

health-related quality of life, 13

heart disease, 10, 76

heart-rate monitors, 159–62

heart rates, 157, 158–62

heat, extreme, 89

height, 92, 94

high-protein diets, 71

hike it up (work out), 154–55

hiking

assessments of, 112

destination planning, 105

equipment and gear for, 88, 101–4

footwear for, 4, 5, 83, 97, 125–26

groups for, 38

hills and speed calculations, 95

as long walks, 81, 85

problem remediation, 111

as strength building, 148

terrain and elements, 95–96

tips for, 96

training for, 96–101

hiking footwear, 4, 5, 83, 97, 125–26

Hill, Jim, 13

hips, exercises for, 42, 210

Hixon, Laney, 144

hockey, field, 174–75

Hot-Furnace Theory, 71

hula-hoop jumps (exercise), 7

ice, as injury remedy, 211

ice dancing, 178

ice sports, 178

injuries

racewalking and, 196–97

walking, 206–12

walking vs. running, 11

instructors, walking, 199

intervals, 153–54

jackets, 55, 104

Journal of the American Medical Association, 13, 60

junk food, 71, 73, 76

kayaking, 173–74

Kent, Kimberly, 176, 177

knapsacks. See backpacks

knees, 79, 85, 208

lacrosse, 174–75

legislation, federal, 235

legs, exercises for, 6, 45, 100, 117, 118, 168, 208, 209

legumes, 77

logs, training

as motivation, 33, 37